Case Studies in Epilepsy

Common and Uncommon Presentations

D1536837

Case Studies in Epilepsy

Common and Uncommon Presentations

Hermann Stefan

Elinor Ben-Menachem

Patrick Chauvel

Renzo Guerrini

WITHDRAWN

TOURO COLLEGE LIBRARY
Midtown

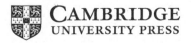

CAMBRIDGE
UNIVERSITY PRESS

MT

CAMBRIDGE UNIVERSITY PRESS
Cambridge, New York, Melbourne, Madrid, Cape Town,
Singapore, São Paulo, Delhi, Mexico City

Cambridge University Press
The Edinburgh Building, Cambridge CB2 8RU, UK

Published in the United States of America by
Cambridge University Press, New York

www.cambridge.org
Information on this title: www.cambridge.org/9780521167123

© Hermann Stefan, Elinor Ben-Menachem, Patrick Chauvel and
Renzo Guerrini 2012

This publication is in copyright. Subject to statutory exception
and to the provisions of relevant collective licensing agreements,
no reproduction of any part may take place without
the written permission of Cambridge University Press.

First published 2012

Printed and bound in the United Kingdom by the MPG Books Group

A catalog record for this publication is available from the British Library

Library of Congress Cataloging-in-Publication Data
Case studies in epilepsy : common and uncommon presentations /
[edited by] Hermann Stefan . . . [et al.].
    p. ; cm.
Includes bibliographical references.
ISBN 978-0-521-16712-3 (Paperback)
I. Stefan, Hermann.
  [DNLM: 1. Epilepsy–diagnosis–Case Reports.   2. Diagnosis,
Differential–Case Reports.   3. Epilepsy–therapy–Case Reports.   WL 385]
616.85′3–dc23

2012021095

ISBN 978-0-521-16712-3 Paperback

Cambridge University Press has no responsibility for the persistence or
accuracy of URLs for external or third-party internet websites referred to
in this publication, and does not guarantee that any content on such
websites is, or will remain, accurate or appropriate.

Every effort has been made in preparing this book to provide accurate and
up-to-date information which is in accord with accepted standards and
practice at the time of publication. Although case histories are drawn from
actual cases, every effort has been made to disguise the identities of the
individuals involved. Nevertheless, the authors, editors and publishers can
make no warranties that the information contained herein is totally free
from error, not least because clinical standards are constantly changing
through research and regulation. The authors, editors and publishers
therefore disclaim all liability for direct or consequential damages resulting
from the use of material contained in this book. Readers are strongly
advised to pay careful attention to information provided by the manufacturer
of any drugs or equipment that they plan to use.

5/28/13

Contents

Section 2 – Treatment

Contributors

Jean-Michel Badier
UMR Inserm U751 & Service de Neurophysiologie Clinique, Faculté de Médecine & Assistance Publique-Hôpitaux de Marseille, Marseille, France

Carmen Barba
Children's Hospital A. Meyer, University of Florence, Firenze, Italy

Yerma Bartolini
Neurology Unit, Bellaria Hospital, IRCCS Institute of Neurological Sciences, Bologna, Italy

Sebastian Bauer
Department of Neurology and Epilepsy Center Hessen, Philipps-University Marburg, Marburg, Germany

Elinor Ben-Menachem
Sahlgren University Hospital, Neurological Department, Göteborg, Sweden

Arnaud Biraben
Service de Neurologie, CHU Pontchaillou, 35000 Rennes, France

Paul Boon
Department of Neurology, Reference Center for Refractory Epilepsy, Institute for Neuroscience, Ghent University Hospital, Belgium

Patrick Chauvel
Faculté de Médecine d'Aix-Marseille Université and Director of the Institut de Neurosciences des Systèmes (INSERM-Universite), Marseille, France

Sophie Colnat-Coulbois
Service de Neurologie, CHU Nancy, 54000 Nancy, France

Alessio De Ciantis
Children's Hospital A. Meyer, University of Florence, Firenze, Italy

Yves Denoyer
Service de Neurologie, CHU Pontchaillou, 35000 Rennes, France

Nathalie Ehrle
Service de Neurologie, CHU Reims, 51000 Reims, France

Melania Falchi
Children's Hospital A. Meyer, University of Florence, Firenze, Italy

Barbara Fiedler
Department of General Pediatrics, University Children's Hospital Münster, Unit Neuropediatrics, Münster, Germany

Stefano Forlivesi
Neurology Unit, Bellaria Hospital, IRCCS Institute of Neurological Sciences, Bologna, Italy

Elena Gardella
Regional Epilepsy Center, University of Milan, San Paolo Hospital, Milan, Italy, and Danish Epilepsy Center, Epilepsihospitalet, Dianalund, Denmark

Martine Gavaret
UMR Inserm U751 & Service de Neurophysiologie Clinique, Faculté de Médecine & Assistance Publique-Hôpitaux de Marseille, Marseille, France

Marco Giulioni
Neurosurgery Unit, Bellaria Hospital, IRCCS Institute of Neurological Sciences, Bologna, Italy

Wolfgang Graf
University Hospital Erlangen, Neurological Clinic – Epilepsy Center, Erlangen, Germany

Renzo Guerrini
Children's Hospital A. Meyer, University of Florence, Firenze, Italy

Thilo Hammen
University Hospital Erlangen, Neurological Clinic –
Epilepsy Center, Erlangen, Germany

Marcel Heers
University Hospital Erlangen, Neurological Clinic –
Epilepsy Center, Erlangen, Germany

Claire Haegelen
Service der Neurochirurgie, CHU Pontchaillou,
35000 Rennes, France

Audrey Henry
Service de Neurologie, CHU Reims, 51000 Reims,
France

Björn Holnberg
Sahlgren University Hospital, Neurological
Department, Göteborg, Sweden

Katrin Hüttemann
University Hospital Erlangen, Neurological Clinic –
Epilepsy Center, Erlangen, Germany

Burkhard Kasper
University Hospital Erlangen, Neurological Clinic –
Epilepsy Center, Erlangen, Germany

Frank Kerling
University Hopsital Erlangen, Neurological Clinic –
Epilepsy Center, Erlangen, Germany

Tobias Knieß
Neurological Clinic, Rhön Klinikum, Bad Neustadt/
Saale, Germany

Gerhard Kurlemann
Department of General Pediatrics, University
Children's Hospital Münster, Unit Neuropediatrics,
Münster, Germany

Nicolas Lang
Adult Epilepsy Center, Department of Neurology,
UKSH Campus Kiel, Germany

Louis Maillard
Service de Neurologie, CHU Nancy, 54000 Nancy,
France

Francesco Mari
Children's Hospital A. Meyer, University of Florence,
Firenze, Italy

Anna Federica Marliani
Neuroradiology Unit, Bellaria Hospital, IRCCS
Institute of Neurological Sciences, Bologna, Italy

Stefano Meletti
Division of Neurology, Department of Neurosciences,
University of Modena and Reggio Emilia, Modena,
Italy

Roberto Michelucci
Neurology Unit, Bellaria Hospital, IRCCS Institute of
Neurological Sciences, Bologna, Italy

Anca Pasnicu
Service d' Explorations Functionelles, CHU
Pontchaillou, 35000 Rennes, France

Elisabeth Pauli
University Hospital Erlangen, Neurological Clinic –
Epilepsy Center, Erlangen, Germany

Jean-Claude Peragut
UMR Inserm U751 & Service de Neurophysiologie
Clinique, Faculté de Médecine & Assistance
Publique-Hôpitaux de Marseille, Marseille, France

Stefan Rampp
University Hospital Erlangen, Neurological Clinic –
Epilepsy Center, Erlangen, Germany

Christophe Rauch
University Hospital Erlangen, Neurological Clinic –
Epilepsy Center, Erlangen, Germany

Felix Rosenow
Department of Neurology and Epilepsy Center Hessen,
Philipps-University Marburg, Marburg, Germany

Guido Rubboli
Neurology Unit, Bellaria Hospital, IRCCS Institute of
Neurological Sciences, Bologna, Italy, and Danish
Epilepsy Center, Epilepsihospitalet, Dianalund,
Denmark

Barbara Schmalbach
Adult Epilepsy Center, Department of Neurology,
UKSH Campus Kiel, Germany

Friedhelm C. Schmitt
University Hospital Magdeburg, Neurological Clinic,
Magdeburg, Germany

Mathieu Sprengers
Department of Neurology, Reference Center for Refractory Epilepsy, Institute for Neuroscience, Ghent University Hospital, Belgium

Hermann Stefan
University Hospital Erlangen, Neurological Clinic – Epilepsy Center, Erlangen, Germany

Adam Strzelczyk
Department of Neurology and Epilepsy Center Hessen, Philipps-University Marburg, Marburg, Germany

Anne Thiriaux
Service de Neurologie, CHU Reims, 51000 Reims, France

Christian Tilz
Krankenhaus Barmherzige Brüder, Neurological Clinic, Linz, Austria, and Krankenhaus 'Barmherzige Brüder', Department of Neurology, Regensburg, Germany

Jean-Pierre Vignal
Service de Neurologie, CHU Nancy, 54000 Nancy, France

Kristl Vonck
Department of Neurology, Reference Center for Refractory Epilepsy, Institute for Neuroscience, Ghent University Hospital, Belgium

Jörg Wellmer
Ruhr-Epileptology, Department of Neurology, University Hospital Knappschaftskrankenhaus, Bochum, Germany

Xintong Wu
University Hospital Erlangen, Neurological Clinic – Epilepsy Center, Erlangen, Germany

Francesco Zellini
Children's Hospital A. Meyer, University of Florence, Firenze, Italy

Preface

Clinical case studies have long been recognized as a useful adjunct to problem-based learning and continuing professional development. They emphasize the need for clinical reasoning, integrative thinking, problem-solving, communication, teamwork, and self-directed learning – all desirable generic skills for health care professionals. Epilepsy is amongst the most frequently encountered of neurological disorders. There are important emerging clinical management issues (e.g., first seizure, therapy-resistant seizures, ICU, pregnancy), but also differential diagnosis of non-epileptic seizures (syncopy, pseudo-seizure, paroxysmal dystonic syndromes, sleep disorders, psychosis, inborn errors of metabolism, etc.). This selection of epilepsy case studies will inform and challenge clinicians at all stages in their careers. Including both common and uncommon cases, *Case Studies in Epilepsy* reinforces the diagnostic skills and treatment decision-making processes necessary to treat epilepsy and other seizures confidently. Written by leading experts, the cases and discussions work through differential diagnoses, treatments, and social consequences in pediatric and adult patients.

The editors collected real-life experiences from epileptologists of different countries. For this purpose, cases were selected to illustrate common and more rare conditions of patients.

The collection of these cases will add practical experiences to more systematic and theoretical-based textbooks of epilepsies providing a systematic overview.

Easy and difficult problems are discussed with regard to the needs of the individual case for a wide range of potential readers in neurology and neuropediatry.

General and special remarks guide the reader through the special requirements of the case and refer to sytematic informations by recommended publications.

I wish to express our gratitude to the co-editors and all the contributors taking the additional burden of writing. I also want to express my thanks to Mrs. Saint-Lôt for her active assistance from the beginning.

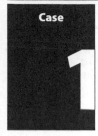

First seizure: is it epilepsy?

Christophe Rauch and Hermann Stefan

History

A 27-year-old man went to a supermarket in the afternoon when he remarked on blurred vision and then lost consciousness. Motoric relinquishings were observed by other customers. The young man regained consciousness upon the arrival of the emergency physician. The physician detected a tongue bite and measured a low blood glucosis level of 45 mg/dl. The patient was referred to the emergency room of the neurological department.

The patient told that this was the first seizure he had suffered. Furthermore, he told that he had not eaten much that day. There were no other diseases known in this patient, no familiar disposition.

Actual treatment

None

What to do?
Further investigations

- **EEG**: Alpha-EEG, no epileptiform activity
- **Blood samples**: Blood glucosis 62 mg/dl, no further noticeable values
- **MRI**: normal finding

Diagnosis

Hypoglycemia with seizure.

Treatment

Treatment of the hypoglycemia and research for reasons for the hypoglycemia. Further investigations for Diabetes mellitus, insulinoma, and further differential diagnosis.

General remarks

According to the consensus definition of seizure and epilepsy by The International League Against Epilepsy (ILAE) and the International Bureau for Epilepsy (IBE), an epileptic seizure is a transient occurrence of signs and/or symptoms due to abnormal excessive or synchronous neuronal activity in the brain.

Special remarks

Hypoglycemia can be one cause for seizures especially if a seizure occurs in the morning before breakfast or after exercise. Therefore, the reason for hypoglycemia needs to be resolved. One misdiagnosis can be an insulinoma which is one of the most common hormone-secreting tumors of the gastrointestinal tract. It causes hypoglycemic phases with symptoms concerning the autonomic system such as sweating, tremor, anxiety, etc. and symptoms concerning the central nerve system such as confusion, lethargy, bizarre behavior, and cognitive troubles, etc. These symptoms can be quite similar to epileptic seizures. Epilepsy can be already diagnosed if only one spontaneous seizure occurs, if signs for an enduring predisposition such as spike-wave activity in the EEG coincide. This was not the case in our patient.

Case Studies in Epilepsy, ed. Hermann Stefan, Elinor Ben-Menachem, Patrick Chauvel and Renzo Guerrini. Published by Cambridge University Press. © Hermann Stefan, Elinor Ben-Menachem, Patrick Chauvel and Renzo Guerrini 2012.

Suggested reading

Fisher RS, van Emde Boas W, Blume W, *et al.* Epileptic seizures and epilepsy: definitions proposed by the International League Against Epilepsy (ILAE) and the International Bureau for Epilepsy (IBE). *Epilepsia* 2005; **46**: 470–2.

Graves TD, Gandhi S, Smith SJM, *et al.* Misdiagnosis of seizures: insulinoma presenting as adult onset seizure disorder.

J Neurol Neurosurg Psychiatry 2004; **75**: 1091–2.

Pohlmann-Eden B, Beghi E, Camfield C, Camfield P. The first seizure and its management in adults and children. *BMJ* 2006; **332**: 339–42.

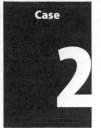

Case

2

Intractable epilepsy and epilepsia partialis continua associated with respiratory chain deficiency

Francesco Mari and Renzo Guerrini

Clinical history

A 5-year-old boy with a history of severe developmental delay and dyskinetic quadriparesis was admitted to our ward after onset of a cluster of convulsive seizures associated with epilepsia partialis continua involving the right facial and shoulder muscles (Fig. 1).

General history

There was no relevant family history of neurological or systemic disorders.

Examination

Dyskinetic quadriparesis. Severe developmental delay. No dysmorphic features.

Image findings

Several brain MRI scans were performed during follow-up. The first scan, 3 days after the admission, showed a left temporo-parieto-occipital ischemic lesion (DWI positive) as well as atrophy brain changes, involving both the cortical and subcortical structures (Fig. 2). A repeat MRI scan, 10 days later, revealed additional ischemic lesions in the frontal lobes.

Follow-up

Epilepsia partialis continua persisted despite treatment with multiple antiepileptic drugs in the intensive care unit. As clinical and brain MRI findings were consistent with a mitochondrial disorder, we performed muscle biopsy.

Special studies

Muscle biopsy with biochemical study of the respiratory chain revealed a deficit of complex I and III activity.

Diagnosis

Mitochondrial encephalopathy (complex I–III deficit) with epilepsia partialis continua.

General remarks

Clinical presentation of respiratory chain defects in childhood causes a large variety of clinical symptoms. In general, a diagnosis of respiratory chain defect is difficult to consider when the initial symptoms occur. Epilepsy is frequently reported with different clinical characteristics including neonatal onset of status epilepticus, Ohtahara syndrome, West syndrome, epilepsia partialis continua, and Alpers syndrome. Appearance of a worsening epileptic syndrome often correlates with a clinically relevant overall worsening of mitochondrial pathology.

Special remarks

Epilepsia partialis continua, i.e., continuous focal jerking involving a body part, is related to a fixed or progressive lesion involving the motor cortex. Several studies have highlighted the relevance of this peculiar epileptic pattern in children with vascular lesions secondary to mitochondrial disorders.

Future perspectives

Despite the increasing knowledge of the molecular bases of mitochondrial encephalomyopathies, no specific treatment for these disorders is available yet. Palliative/supportive measures and metabolic therapies are useful in ameliorating specific problems and quality of life of patients. Gene therapy is a promising approach, but the clinical relevance of its use remains elusive.

Case Studies in Epilepsy, ed. Hermann Stefan, Elinor Ben-Menachem, Patrick Chauvel and Renzo Guerrini. Published by Cambridge University Press. © Hermann Stefan, Elinor Ben-Menachem, Patrick Chauvel and Renzo Guerrini 2012.

(a)

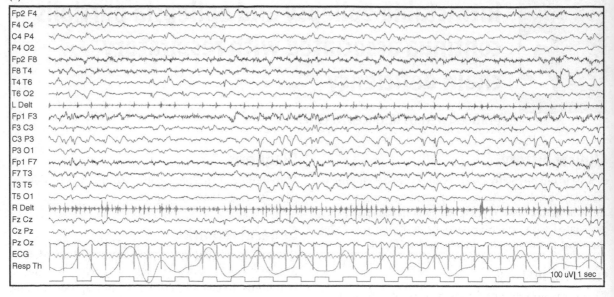

(b)

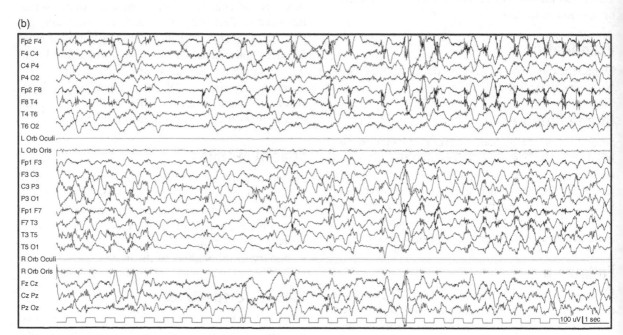

Fig. 1(a), (b). Polygraphic video–EEG recordings: diffusely slow background activity with superimposed rhythmic spikes and slow-waves over the left hemisphere, with centro-parietal predominance. Continuous myoclonic potentials are recorded over the right deltoid and also involve the right orbicularis oris.

(a)

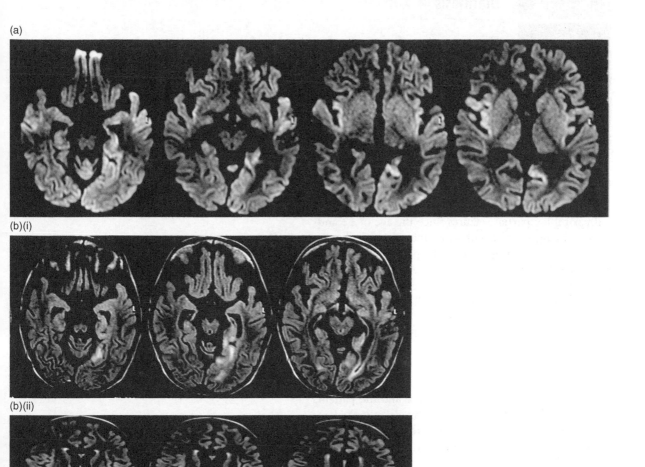

(b)(i)

(b)(ii)

Fig. 2. Axial brain MRI images (a) DWI and (b) FLAIR: subacute left temporo-occipital vascular lesion and mild diffuse cortical and subcortical atrophy.

Suggested reading

Cockerell OC, Rothwell J, Thompson PD, Marsden CD, Shorvon SD. Clinical and physiological features of epilepsia partialis continua. Cases ascertained in the UK. *Brain* 1996; **119**: 393–407.

DiMauro S, Schon EA. Mitochondrial respiratory-chain diseases. *N Engl J Med* 2003; **348**: 2656–68.

Riquet A, Auvin S, Cuisset JM, *et al*. Epilepsia partialis continua and defects in the mitochondrial respiratory chain. *Epilepsy Res* 2008; **78**: 1–6.

Sabbagh SE, Lebre A, Bahi-Buisson N, *et al*. Epileptic phenotypes in children with respiratory chain disorders. *Epilepsia* 2010; **51**: 1225–35.

Veggiotti P, Colamaria V, Dalla Bernardina B, *et al*. Epilepsia partialis continua in a case of MELAS: clinical and neurophysiological study. *Neurophysiol Clin* 1995; **25**: 158–66.

Reasons for violent behavior – when a man strangles his wife

Frank Kerling and Hermann Stefan

Clinical history

A 44-year-old patient was suffering from epilepsy with complex partial seizures since the age of 12 and he was being treated with ethosuximide and pheny-toin. Under this drug regimen the patient was seizure free during day-time, but there were nocturnal episodes of walking around, opening/closing doors and afterwards falling asleep again. The patient had no memory of the event and his wife reported that her husband was not reacting when she talked to him. One night she tried to hold him, because he wanted to leave the house. In this situation he tried to strangle her and she and her daughter were extremely scared. Therefore she thought about divorce and the patient had to sleep in the cellar with the door locked at night-time. He was very desperate and remorseful because of the situation and was admitted to our hospital for diagnostic reasons.

Examination

Neurological and psychiatric examinations were without any pathological findings except for a somehow depressed mood because of the familial situation.

Special studies

In video-EEG monitoring one nocturnal complex-partial seizure was detected. The patient showed nose wiping, oral automatisms, rocking body movements, and an increased muscle tone in the right face and arm. Initially, there was a right frontotemporal 6 Hz pattern and after 34 seconds the pattern propagated to the left temporal lobe. The seizure was followed by a 15-minute state of confusion, wandering, and aggressiveness. Afterwards, the patient was not able to remember the seizure or the confusion. MRI was normal and interictal SPECT showed hypoperfusion left temporal.

Follow-up

We informed the patient and his wife that he was suffering from nocturnal seizures and that the violence was due to postictal confusion. Therefore, we optimized pharmacotherapy and started a new combination with oxcarbazepine and levetiracetam. Ethosuximide and phenytoin therapy were stopped or tapered down, respectively. The patient was almost seizure free with one seizure every 6 months and the patient and his family were satisfied with this result.

Diagnosis

Postictal confusion with aggressive behavior.

General remarks

Postictal aggression and violence against others are pretty rare with a percentage from 5% to 10% of all postictal confusional states. There is clinical heterogeneity among patients with postictal violence with respect to etiology of epilepsy, age of onset, laterality, and memory of adverse behaviors. Several clinical features, including male gender, are common. Typically, the episodes of postictal aggression are not isolated events, but recur repeatedly often with stereotyped behaviors. Subacute postictal aggression is even more likely after a cluster of seizures than after a single ictus. Aggression occurs especially when relatives or hospital staff try to restrain the patient. Most of the patients have medically intractable epilepsy and are remorseful in the interictal period like our patient was.

Case Studies in Epilepsy, ed. Hermann Stefan, Elinor Ben-Menachem, Patrick Chauvel and Renzo Guerrini. Published by Cambridge University Press. © Hermann Stefan, Elinor Ben-Menachem, Patrick Chauvel and Renzo Guerrini 2012.

Special remarks

Our patient showed abnormal violence during a typical state of nocturnal confusion, when his wife tried to restrain him. He had been suffering from epilepsy for decades and was seizure free during the day-time. A postictal aggression was more probable than somnambulism. There is evidence that nocturnal seizures, especially without tonic–clonic movements, can be missed by the partner and only the confusion is noticed. The results of the video–EEG helped the patient and his family to understand the context between seizures and confusion and the familial situation was stabilized. A modified drug therapy led to sufficient seizure control.

Suggested reading

Gerard ME, Spitz MC, Towbin JA, Shantz D. Subacute postictal aggression. *Neurology* 1998; **50**: 384–8.

Ito M, Okazaki M, Takahashi S, *et al.* Subacute postictal aggression in patients with epilepsy. *Epilepsy Behav* 2007; **10**: 611–14.

Marsh L, Krauss GL. Aggression and violence in patients with epilepsy. *Epilepsy Behav* 2000; **1**: 160–8.

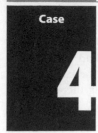

4

Repetitive monocular eye adduction

Adam Strzelczyk, Sebastian Bauer, and Felix Rosenow

Clinical history

A 24-year-old student presented with recurring episodes of involuntary eye movements without disturbance of consciousness for the last 3 weeks. He reported suffering from 5 to 8 attacks per day with an initial feeling of slightly impaired vision followed by adduction of the left eye only lasting for up to 10 seconds. For the last 5 days he had also noticed hypoesthesia of the left hand during these episodes. For that reason, he presented to the neurological emergency department.

Examination

At the physical, neurological, and ophthalmologic examination including visual fields, no abnormalities were detected. He had no history of febrile convulsions, seizures, or any other risk factors for epilepsy. An episode as described above was observed by the treating physician and an EEG with video recording was recommended.

Special studies

During a 2-hour video–EEG monitoring two right frontal EEG seizures (max. F4/C4) of up to 17 seconds duration were recorded, all of which were accompanied by an adduction of the left eye and symmetrical head nodding. No other ictal or postictal symptoms were observed. Visual evoked potentials were within normal limits (Fig. 1a,b).

Image findings

3T MRI sagittal FLAIR images showed a right frontal focal cortical dysplasia. No other focal lesions were detected (Fig. 2).

Follow-up

Initial treatment with levetiracetam up to 4000 mg daily led to a decrease in seizure frequency by half. With a change of anticonvulsive treatment to carbamazepine 400 mg daily, a sustained seizure freedom of more than 2 years could be achieved.

Diagnosis

Symptomatic focal right frontal epilepsy.

Seizures:	simple motor seizures -> somatosensory auras
Cause:	right frontal cortical dysplasia
Related medical conditions:	none

General remarks

Monocular nystagmus is a rare and heterogenous neurological phenomenon. It is usually not of epileptic origin and has been reported in cases of anterior visual pathway lesions, monocular blindness, spasmus nutans, and brainstem lesions associated with stroke or multiple sclerosis. Epileptic binocular nystagmus remains also an infrequent semiological finding and should not be confused with the epileptic gaze deviation. The physiology of binocular epileptic nystagmus is incompletely understood. Kaplan and colleagues postulated that epileptic nystagmus is mediated by a seizure focus in a cortical saccade region contraversive to both quick and slow phases of nystagmus.

Grant and colleagues reported a case of epileptic monocular nystagmus with seizures originating in the

Case Studies in Epilepsy, ed. Hermann Stefan, Elinor Ben-Menachem, Patrick Chauvel and Renzo Guerrini. Published by Cambridge University Press. © Hermann Stefan, Elinor Ben-Menachem, Patrick Chauvel and Renzo Guerrini 2012.

(a)

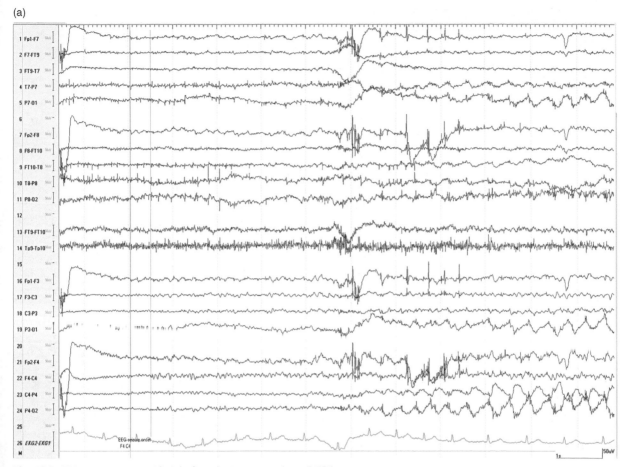

Fig. 1(a). EEG seizure pattern with right frontal seizure onset (max. F4/C4).

occipital lobe, pointing towards an activated cortical saccade region, which caused simultaneous supranuclear inhibition of ipsilateral eye movement or triggered monocular eye movement commands. Both our case and the one reported by Grant are at variance with Hering's law, which postulated that premotor eye movement commands are always binocular, and that these commands consist of separate components for the control of saccades and accommodation.

Special remarks

Recent data from invasive video–EEG monitoring with subdural grids reported by Thurtell and colleagues give evidence for a three-dimensional cortical control of gaze mediated by the frontal eye fields. Based on earlier findings from lesion, imaging, and stimulation studies the human frontal eye fields are thought to be located at the caudal end of the middle frontal gyrus known to be in control of contralateral versive eye movements, saccades, and smooth pursuit.

Both described patients developed disconjugated contraversive horizontal eye movements in response to electrical stimulation of the frontal cortex or during focal seizures close to the frontal eye field.

Suggested reading

Grant AC, Jain V, Bose S, *et al.* 'Epileptic monocular nystagmus'. *Neurology* 2002; **59**: 1438–41.

Kaplan PW, Tusa RJ. 'Neurophysiologic and clinical correlations of epileptic nystagmus'. *Neurology* 1993; **43**: 2508–14.

Lobel E, Kahane P, Leonardis U, *et al.* 'Localization of human frontal eye fields: anatomical and functional findings of functional magnetic resonance imaging and intracerebral

(b)

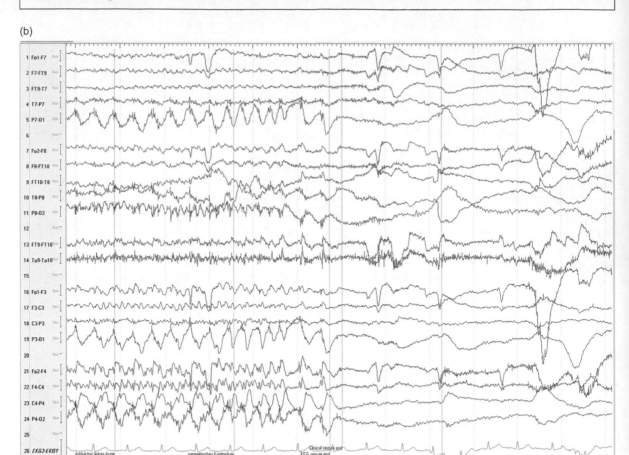

Fig. 1(b). Right frontal EEG seizure pattern; please note the occipital artifacts due to symmetrical head nodding.

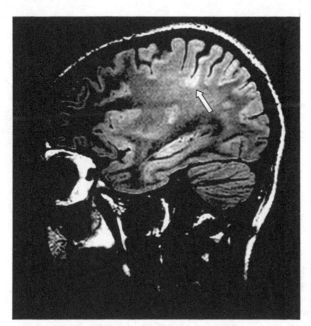

Fig. 2. Sagittal FLAIR image with a right frontal focal cortical dysplasia (arrow).

electrical stimulation'. *J Neurosurg* 2001; **95**: 804–15.

Lüders H, Acharya J, Baumgartner C, *et al.* Semiological seizure classification. *Epilepsia* 1998; **39**: 1006–13.

Thurtell MJ, Mohamed A, Lüders HO, Leigh RJ. 'Evidence for three-dimensional cortical control of gaze from epileptic patients'. *J Neurol Neurosurg Psychiatry* 2009; **80**: 683–5.

Yee RD, Jelks GW, Baloh RW, Honniba V. Uniocular nystagmus in monocular visual loss. *Ophthalmology* 1979; **86**: 511–22.

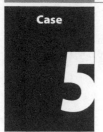

Febrile infectious-related epilepsy syndrome (FIRES)

Francesco Zellini and Renzo Guerrini

Clinical history

A 14-year-old girl with normal psychomotor development was admitted to our hospital with convulsive status epilepticus.

Focal seizures rapidly evolving into status epilepticus had appeared, without fever, about 10 days after a non-specific upper respiratory tract infection. Progressive spread of seizures arising independently from either side of the body produced secondary generalization.

Family history

No family history of neuropsychiatric conditions.

Neurological examination

Patient was intubated and markedly sedated. GCS: 9.

Special studies

Several seizures starting independently from either the left or right frontal temporal region were recorded during video–EEG. Brain MRI and CSF study were unrevealing.

Follow-up

Status epilepticus was refractory to multiple treatments. Burst-suppression coma was achieved using general anesthesia in the intensive care unit. After status epilepticus subsided, the patient experienced a 2 month seizure-free period, after which focal epilepsy developed, with sporadic secondarily generalized seizures. In the following 4 years an average of two seizures per year occurred. Neuropsychological testing revealed impaired executive functions.

Diagnosis

Febrile infectious-related epilepsy syndrome (FIRES).

General remarks

Febrile infection-related epilepsy syndrome is an increasingly recognized epilepsy entity that presents with multifocal refractory status epilepticus in previously healthy school-aged children. It starts abruptly a few days to 1 week after a non-specific febrile illness. Children manifest seizures that rapidly worsen and translate into status epilepticus. This acute phase is often followed, without an intervening silent period, by a chronic phase characterized by pharmacoresistant epilepsy and severely impaired cognition. An immunological or infective pathogenesis was postulated, but not confirmed by CSF studies. Brain MRI is usually normal in the acute phase, leading to moderate to severe atrophy. Cortical and subcortical T2 high signal intensity abnormalities are at times found a few weeks after onset, possibly related to cytotoxic edema. The absence of inflammatory markers (including no histologic evidence of inflammation reported on brain biopsy or postmortem specimens), and the poor response to immunomodulating or immunosuppressant treatments make the diagnosis of encephalitis inappropriate, and suggest FIRES to be best conceptualized as chronic epilepsy with an explosive onset.

Special remarks

Despite a prolonged acute phase with refractory status epilepticus leading to intensive care unit management, cognitive outcome was relatively

Case Studies in Epilepsy, ed. Hermann Stefan, Elinor Ben-Menachem, Patrick Chauvel and Renzo Guerrini. Published by Cambridge University Press. © Hermann Stefan, Elinor Ben-Menachem, Patrick Chauvel and Renzo Guerrini 2012.

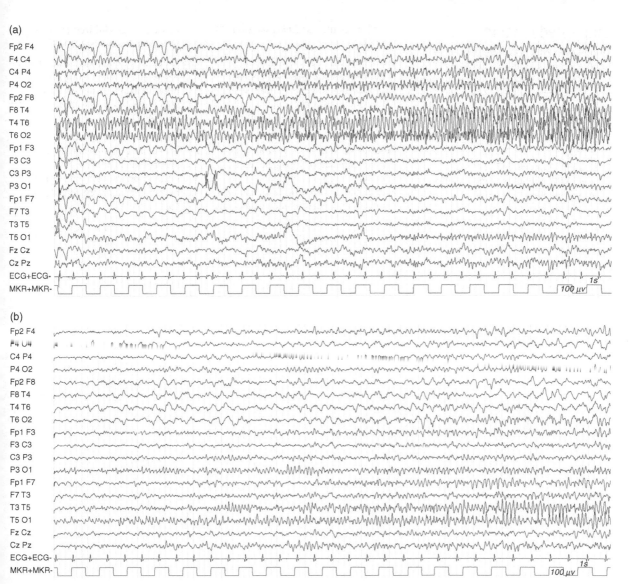

Fig. 1. EEG recording showing focal seizure activity arising from either hemisphere. Both seizures, which were hours apart, were followed by secondary generalization.

good in this patient. Follow-up MRI showed mild global atrophy. Several attempts to reduce AED polytherapy were followed by relapse of seizures, revealing a condition of pharmacodependency.

Future perspectives

An association with elevated voltage-gated potassium channel (VGKC) complex antibodies and a significant clinical and immunological response to immunomodulation was recently reported in a patient with FIRES. Although extensive neuronal surface antibodies investigation is usually negative in these patients, a considerable effort should be devoted to searching for potentially treatable conditions. A better understanding of the pathogenic mechanisms triggering FIRES might increase the chances of devising a more effective treatment strategy in the acute phase, hopefully minimizing the long-term cognitive sequelae of this ominous and mysterious condition (Fig. 1).

Suggested reading

Illingworth MA, Hanrahan D, Anderson CE, *et al.* Elevated VGKC-complex antibodies in a boy with fever-induced refractory epileptic encephalopathy in school-age children (FIRES). *Dev Med Child Neurol* 2011; 53: 1053–7.

Ismail FY, Kossoff EH. AERRPS, DESC, NORSE, FIRES: multi-labeling or distinct epileptic entities? *Epilepsia* 2011; 52: e185–9.

Kramer U, Chi CS, Lin KL, *et al.* Febrile infection-related epilepsy syndrome (FIRES): pathogenesis, treatment, and outcome: a multicenter study on 77 children. *Epilepsia* 2011; 52: 1956–65.

Nabbout R, Mazzuca M, Hubert P, *et al.* Efficacy of ketogenic diet in severe refractory status epilepticus initiating fever induced refractory epileptic encephalopathy in school age children (FIRES). *Epilepsia* 2010; 51: 2033–7.

Nabbout R, Vezzani A, Dulac O, *et al.* Acute encephalopathy with inflammation-mediated status epilepticus. *Lancet Neurol* 2011; 10: 99–108.

van Baalen A, Häusler M, Boor R, *et al.* Febrile infection-related epilepsy syndrome (FIRES): a nonencephalitic encephalopathy in childhood. *Epilepsia* 2010; 51: 1323–8.

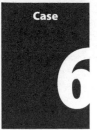

Case

6

Epileptic seizures as presenting symptom of the shaken baby syndrome

Alessio De Ciantis and Renzo Guerrini

Clinical history

A 5-month-old boy, born at term after normal delivery, was admitted after onset of focal seizures with secondary generalization. He appeared to be drowsy. The parents reported that the child had lost consciousness after bumping his head on a baby chair and that his father had immediately shaken the boy with the intent of bringing him back to consciousness.

Examination

On initial evaluation, the child was alert and responsive, with no neurological signs.

Special studies

Routine laboratory investigations were normal. Computerized tomography (CT) of the brain showed acute subdural hematomas along the posterior cerebral falx and posterior fossa and in the posterior surface of the occipital lobes (Fig.1 a,b). Phenobarbital was introduced, with consequent control of generalized seizures, but persistence of subclinical multifocal seizure activity on the EEG.

Follow-up

Brain magnetic resonance imaging (MRI), performed 4 days later, revealed extensive areas of low intensity signal of the cortex and white matter in the frontal and temporal lobes (Fig. 2b). Extensive restriction of diffusion in the white matter, suggestive of severe ischemia, was seen using diffusion-weighted sequences (Fig. 2a). Ophthalmologic examination revealed retinal hemorrhages confined to the posterior pole and rare flame-shaped hemorrhages. Video–EEG monitoring on the fifth day after onset of symptoms demonstrated alternating ictal activity originating from either the left or the right fronto-centro-temporal area, without any clinical symptoms (Fig. 3a,b). Due to persisting seizure, activity carbamazepine was introduced, which terminated seizures. Follow-up MRI, 17 days later, showed residual left hemispheric and basal occipital hematomas, with recent internal bleedings and subcortical atrophy (Fig. 2c). Therefore the hematoma was drained and a subdural-peritoneal shunt placement was performed. Two months after admission, the boy was discharged from hospital with a clinical picture including spastic quadriparesis, defective eye tracking, irritability, and impaired social interaction and communication.

Image findings (Figs. 1, 2)

EEG findings (Fig. 3)

Diagnosis

Shaken Baby syndrome.

General remarks

Shaken Baby syndrome (SBS) is a form of inflicted head trauma. SBS may be misdiagnosed and underdiagnosed, and caregivers may lie or be unaware of the mechanism of injury. The injuries associated with SBS may not be immediately noticeable. A shaken child may present non-specific symptoms such as lethargy, irritability, vomiting, or major neurological changes such as seizures, coma, or stupor. This condition is often diagnosed based on finding subdural and retinal hemorrhages in infants referred for

Case Studies in Epilepsy, ed. Hermann Stefan, Elinor Ben-Menachem, Patrick Chauvel and Renzo Guerrini. Published by Cambridge University Press. © Hermann Stefan, Elinor Ben-Menachem, Patrick Chauvel and Renzo Guerrini 2012.

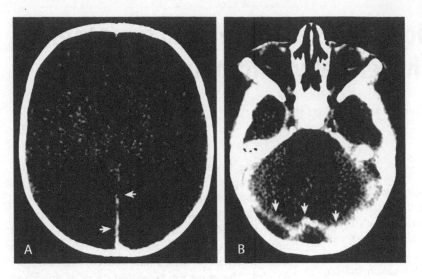

Fig. 1. Axial brain CT scan, performed 48 hours after the onset of symptoms, showing acute subdural hematomas along the posterior cerebral falx (A, arrows), the posterior surfaces of the occipital lobes and the posterior fossa (B, arrows).

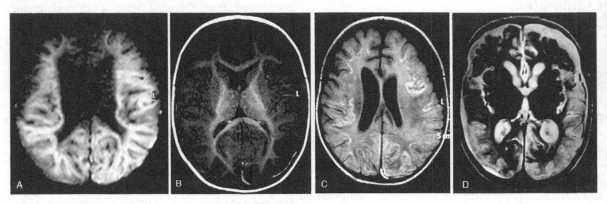

Fig. 2. A. Axial DWI MR, performed 4 days after onset of symptoms. There is an extensive bilateral hemispheric restricted diffusion, corresponding to severe ischemia, with a drop in the apparent diffusion coefficient (ADC). B. Axial T1WI MR, performed at the same time as the above DWI, shows extensive low intensity in the white matter. C. Follow-up axial T2 FLAIR sense, performed 17 days after A and B, shows residual left hemispheric and basal occipital hematomas, with recent internal bleedings and subcortical atrophy. D. Follow-up axial T2WI MRI performed 37 days after A, B. There is diffuse brain atrophy with high intensity abnormalities in the cerebral cortex and white matter, cortical thinning, and multiple subdural collections of different signal intensities and ages.

seemingly new onset seizures or "de novo" status epilepticus (SE) and no history of trauma. Children with SBS do not typically present with a lucid interval, they become symptomatic, most often losing consciousness, immediately after the abusive head trauma. Infants and small children are especially vulnerable to head injuries because of the unique anatomical features of their head and brain. The majority of victims are infants aged less than 1 year, although these injuries can be seen in children up to 5 years old. There is equal gender distribution with slight male predominance. The perpetrators are most often parents or caregivers. The estimated mortality rate ranges from 13% to 30% and the increase of intracranial pressure secondary to brain swelling is the most frequent cause of death. Up to 50% of survivors suffer permanent cognitive or other neurological disability, and 30% have a chance for full recovery.

Special remarks

Post-traumatic seizures (PTS) occur more frequently in children with inflicted (65%–74%) vs. non-inflicted traumatic brain injury (15%–17%).

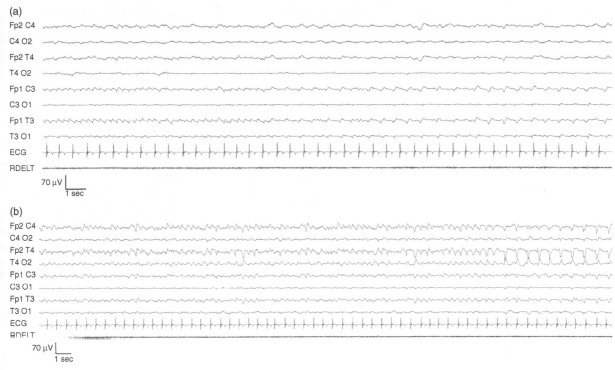

Fig. 3. EEG recording performed 6 days after onset of symptoms. At the time of recording, the boy was drowsy and irritable but no clinically overt seizure activity was apparent. In (a) ictal activity originating from the left fronto-centro-temporal area. In (b) a few minutes later, there is ictal electrographic activity over the homologous contralateral region.

They are classified as immediate (within 24 hours after the injury), early (between 24 hours and a week) or late (after longer than 1 week following the trauma). Immediate and early PTS are thought to result from a direct reaction to the injury (direct neurologic or systemic effects of head trauma), while late seizures result from permanent structural changes in the brain. Immediate seizures, which make up to 50%–80% of early seizures, are particularly frequent after severe traumatic brain injury. Seizures consequent to SBS are of different semiology, including generalized tonic–clonic, unilateral, or focal. Multiple foci of cerebral injury may manifest with more than one seizure type. Appearance of seizures is associated with an unfavorable neurodevelopmental outcome. Status epilepticus is most often observed in children with severe injury and represents the greatest risk of adverse outcome.

Sub-clinical SE was identified in 25% of children with SBS. Various drugs have been used with the purpose of preventing seizures and epilepsy in SBS, but antiepileptic drug prophylaxis of PTS is still a controversial issue. It is recommended that PTS be treated as one would treat seizures of the same type of any etiology. The same rule applies to the medical treatment of SE occurring at any time after SBS.

Future perspectives

Crying and irritation of children are common causes of frustration that can induce impulsive and harmful action in care givers. In order to prevent SBS, it is therefore vitally important to educate new parents, babysitters and anyone handling babies and small children never ever to shake them, under any circumstance.

Suggested reading

Adelson PD, Bratton SL, Carney NA, et al. American Association for Surgery of Trauma; Child Neurology Society; International Society for Pediatric Neurosurgery; International Trauma Anesthesia and Critical Care Society; Society of Critical Care Medicine; World Federation of Pediatric Intensive and Critical Care Societies. Guidelines for the acute medical management of severe traumatic brain injury in infants, children, and adolescents. Chapter 19. The role of anti-seizure prophylaxis following severe pediatric traumatic brain injury. *Pediatr Crit. Care Med* 2003; **4**: S72–5.

Barlow KM, Spowart JJ, Minns RA. Early posttraumatic seizures in non-accidental head injury: relation to outcome. *Dev Med Child Neurol* 2000; **42**: 591–4.

Blumenthal I. Shaken baby syndrome. *Postgrad Med J* 2002; **78**: 732–5.

Bourgeois M, Di Rocco F, Garnett M, *et al*. Epilepsy associated with shaken baby syndrome. *Childs Nerv Syst* 2008; **24**: 169–72.

Duhaime AC, Durham S. Traumatic brain injury in infants: the phenomenon of subdural hemorrhage with hemispheric hypodensity ("Big Black Brain").

Prog Brain Res 2007; **161**: 293–302.

Ewing-Cobbs L, Prasad M, Kramer L, *et al*. Acute neuroradiologic findings in young children with inflicted or noninflicted traumatic brain injury. *Childs Nerv Syst* 2000; **16**: 25–33.

Facco E. Current topics. The role of EEG in brain injury. *Intens Care Med* 1999; **25**: 872–7.

Guerrini R, De Ciantis A. Non accidental brain injury. In SD Shorvon, F Andermann, R Guerrini, eds. *The Causes of Epilepsy*. Cambridge: Cambridge University Press, 2011, 425–32.

Langendorf FG, Pedley TA, Temkin NR. Posttraumatic seizures. In J Engel Jr, TA Pedley (eds). *Epilepsy: A Comprehensive Textbook*.

Philadelphia, PA: Lippincott Williams & Wilkins, 2008, 2537–42.

Ratan SK, Kulshreshtha R, Pandey RM. Predictors of posttraumatic convulsions in head-injured children. *Pediatr Neurosurg* 1999; **30**: 127–31.

Squier W. The "Shaken Baby" syndrome: pathology and mechanisms. *Acta Neuropathol* 2011; **122**: 519–42.

Stoodley N. Neuroimaging in non-accidental head injury: if, when, why and how. *Clin Radiol*. 2005; **60**: 22–30.

Togioka BM, Arnold MA, Bathurst MA, *et al*. Retinal hemorrhages and shaken baby syndrome: an evidence-based review. *J Emerg Med* 2009; **37**: 98–106.

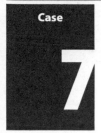

Benign rolandic epilepsy

Francesco Mari and Renzo Guerrini

Clinical history

A 5-year-old girl patient was brought to our attention after a single focal motor seizure that had appeared on awakening, involving the orbicularis oris muscles on the right accompanied by drooling and vomiting.

General history

The child's mother had experienced a single febrile seizure at age 7 years.

Examination

Neurological examination and cognitive testing were normal. EEG showed normal background activity with frequent spikes over the right central region, greatly activated during sleep.

Image findings

Brain MRI was normal.

Follow-up

Rare, brief focal motor seizures alternately involving the muscles of either side of the face were subsequently reported, always appearing within the first 30 minutes after falling asleep. EEG recordings showed bilateral synchronous and asynchronous spikes over centro-temporal regions (Figs. 1 and 2).

Diagnosis

Benign Childhood Epilepsy with Centro-Temporal Spikes (BCECTS), or benign rolandic epilepsy.

General remarks

Benign rolandic epilepsy is one of the most common childhood epilepsy syndromes, occurring in 15%–20% of pediatric epilepsy patients. Seizures begin in middle childhood and resolve by puberty. The total number of seizures experienced by every patient is highly variable, with some only having a few and others presenting dozens of attacks at times concentrated within short periods of time intercalated with long remissions. Interictal EEG is highly distinctive, showing centro-temporal spikes that are typically activated during sleep. The benign evolution of the syndrome can be predicted from the time of diagnosis. Therapy can be withheld in most patients, since seizures are relatively rare and harmless. There is no evidence that drug treatment is actually beneficial, but it may be considered in children exhibiting secondarily generalized seizures.

Special remarks

There are atypical presentations of BCECTS, whose prognosis is not benign, as seizures may be difficult to treat, atonic seizures and severe epileptiform discharges during sleep may appear, and learning difficulties are frequently observed.

Future perspectives

A genetic predisposition with simple or complex modes of inheritance has long been suspected in rolandic epilepsy (Rudolf *et al.*, 2009). However, twin studies showed the absence of any concordant twin pairs with rolandic epilepsy, suggesting a minor role for genetic factors in these patients (Vadlamudi *et al.*, 2006).

Case Studies in Epilepsy, ed. Hermann Stefan, Elinor Ben-Menachem, Patrick Chauvel and Renzo Guerrini. Published by Cambridge University Press. © Hermann Stefan, Elinor Ben-Menachem, Patrick Chauvel and Renzo Guerrini 2012.

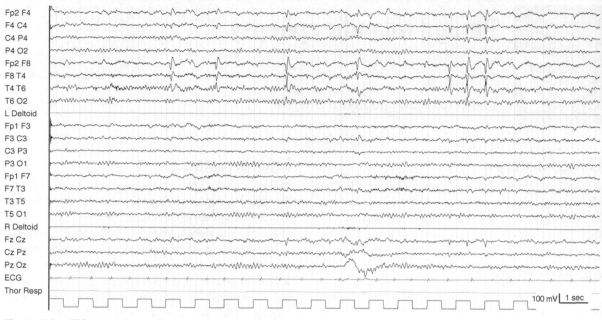

Fig. 1. Video–EEG recorded soon after awakening: normal background, diphasic spikes over right centro-temporal region.

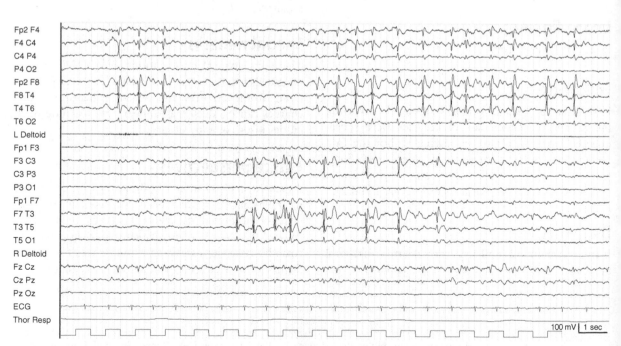

Fig. 2. Video–EEG during slow-wave sleep: activation of bilateral and asynchronous diphasic spikes.

Suggested reading

Fejerman N. Atypical rolandic epilepsy. *Epilepsia* 2009; **50**: 9–12.

Oguni H. Treatment of benign focal epilepsies in children: when and how should be treated? *Brain Dev* 2011; **33**: 207–12.

Rudolf G, Valenti MP, Hirsch E, Szepetowski P. From rolandic epilepsy to continuous spike-and-waves during sleep and Landau–Kleffner syndromes: insights into possible genetic factors. *Epilepsia* 2009; **50**: 25–8.

Shields WD, Snead OC 3rd. Benign epilepsy with centrotemporal spikes. *Epilepsia* 2009; **50**: 10–15.

Vadlamudi L, Kjeldsen MJ, Corey LA, *et al.* Analysing the etiology of benign rolandic epilepsy: a multicentre twin collaboration. *Epilepsia* 2006; **47**: 550–5.

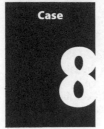

Case

8

New onset focal and generalized epilepsy in an elderly patient

Adam Strzelczyk and Felix Rosenow

Clinical history

A 52-year-old lady with Down syndrome and dementia onset 2 years prior to presentation came as an outpatient for a second opinion.

She had suffered from cerebral ischemia of the left middle cerebral artery 1 year ago and a first generalized tonic–clonic seizure (GTCS) occurred 1 month after that. The diagnosis of post-stroke epilepsy was established at that time and she was started on carbamazepine 300 mg daily. Despite anticonvulsive treatment, she had continued to have one GTCS per month for the last 10 months. Her condition worsened further as she developed disabling myoclonic jerks, which occurred daily and were frequently associated with falls.

Examination

On clinical evaluation, physical characteristics of Down syndrome as epicanthic folds, macroglossia, flat nasal bridge, and a single palmar crease were present. The neurological examination revealed mild right-sided brachiofacial hemiparesis, moderate to severe dementia with reduced speech production, and myoclonic jerks in all four limbs. The patient had no history of febrile convulsions or any other risk factors for epilepsy.

Special studies

During a routine EEG session, continuous generalized slowing, left fronto-temporal sharp waves (maximum F7), and generalized polyspikes were recorded. One generalized tonic–clonic seizure of 80 seconds was recorded during photic stimulation with bioccipital onset.

Image findings (Figs. 1, 2)

Computed axial tomography (CT) was performed while the patient presented with stroke symptoms.

The images showed an infarct anterior and superior of suspected Broca's area in the territory of the left middle cerebral artery (MCA). Please note the general cortical atrophy with enlarged ventricles.

Follow-up

Anticonvulsant treatment with carbamazepine was discontinued and levetiracetam was titrated up to 2000 mg daily. On that regimen the patient stayed free of myoclonus and GTCS for a period of 8 months. Myoclonus then reappeared and levetiracetam was successively increased to 4500 mg daily, resulting in a marked decrease of myoclonus. Upon GTCS reoccurence, valproate was administered as an add-on therapy. However, valproate had to be discontinued due to development of encephalopathy.

Diagnosis

Symptomatic focal left temporo-frontal post-stroke epilepsy and late-onset myoclonic epilepsy in Down syndrome (LOMEDS).

Seizures	Myoclonus
	Generalized tonic–clonic seizures
Cause	Left-sided MCA stroke
	Down syndrome
Related medical conditions	Dementia
	Right-sided hemiparesis
	Hypothyroidism

Case Studies in Epilepsy, ed. Hermann Stefan, Elinor Ben-Menachem, Patrick Chauvel and Renzo Guerrini. Published by Cambridge University Press. © Hermann Stefan, Elinor Ben-Menachem, Patrick Chauvel and Renzo Guerrini 2012.

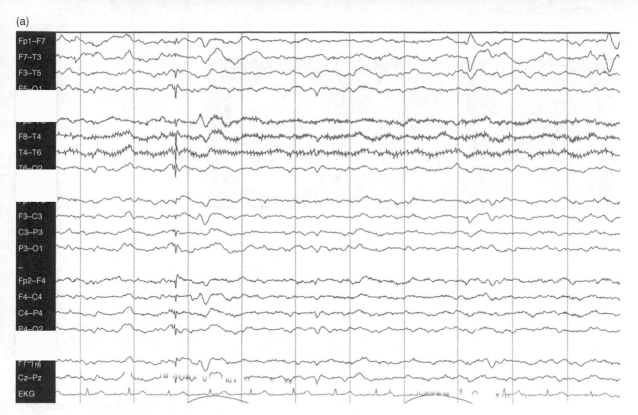

Fig. 1(a). Continuous generalized slowing, left frontotemporal sharp waves (maximum F7) and generalized polyspikes.

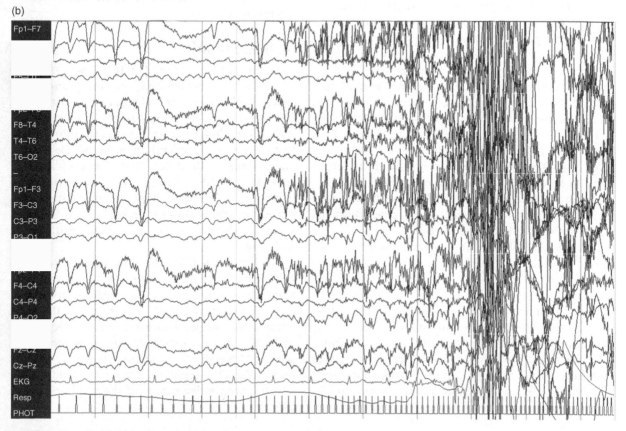

Fig. 1(b). EEG seizure pattern, biooccipital onset during photic stimulation (max O1/O2).

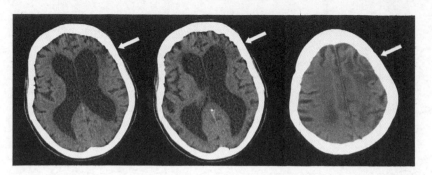

Fig. 2. Axial CCT with general cortical atrophy and enlarged ventricles. Signs of cerebral infarction (arrows) are present in the territory of the left middle cerebral artery (MCA).

General remarks

Although seizures and epilepsy were not mentioned in the original description of Down syndrome (DS), the prevalence in this patient group is now known to be higher than in the general population and increases markedly with age. Seizures in patients with DS are recognized as a significant cause of additional handicap and morbidity, while approximately 9% of patients have epilepsy by the age of 18 years and 46% over the age of 50 years. A triphasic distribution of seizure onset has been discussed, with a first peak incidence during early childhood, the second in early adulthood, and a distinct epilepsy syndrome associated with progressive dementia, myoclonus and GTCS in patients around the age of 50 years. Usually, the onset of cognitive deterioration precedes the onset of myoclonus and GTCS by 1 to 2 years in these patient groups. The terms late-onset myoclonic epilepsy in Down syndrome (LOMEDS) and senile myoclonic epilepsy have been coined for this syndrome. Due to growing life expectancy in individuals with DS, the neurologist will face an increasing proportion of elderly with LOMEDS in future.

In the general population seizures secondary to cerebrovascular disease have been recognized as a major cause of epilepsy in the elderly. Post-stroke epilepsy represents more than 45% of all incident cases aged above 60 years and cerebrovascular disease overall is the cause for around 11% of all epilepsies. Studies described different risk factors for the development of recurrent post-stroke seizures such as hemorrhagic stroke, cortical involvement, large infarction, stroke severity, acute confusional state, and vascular encephalopathy. The

Oxfordshire community stroke project estimated the probability of having a post-stroke seizure at 5.7% within 1 year and averaged a further incremental risk of about 1.5% per year for a total follow-up of 5 years.

Our patient had several predisposing factors for the development of both post-stroke epilepsy and LOMEDS. Obviously, treatment with carbamazepine could only address one of the etiologies and a switch to a broad-spectrum anticonvulsant agent was the treatment of choice.

Special remarks

EEG in patients with LOMEDS will typically show diffuse generalized slowing, generalized spikes, spike-waves, or polyspike-wave complexes. The association of polyspike-wave complexes preceding myoclonus allows the classification of primary generalized epileptic myoclonus. De Simone and colleagues described that 6 out of their 17 patients (35%) showed a photoparoxysmal response on intermittent photic stimulation consisting of brief myoclonic jerks. In their study no patient exhibited signs of photosensitivity in daily life.

Patients with LOMEDS will benefit from anticonvulsive treatment. Levetiracetam and valproate, alone or in combination, may prevent myoclonus as well as seizures and appear to be the most efficacious. Further treatment options are topiramate, lamotrigine, piracetam, and possibly zonisamide. Although the patients respond well to anticonvulsants, cognition usually tends to decline and the progressive course of the condition is not altered.

Suggested reading

Burn J, Dennis M, Bamford J, *et al.* Epileptic seizures after a first stroke: the Oxfordshire Community Stroke Project. *BMJ* 1997; **315**: 1582–7.

De Simone R, Puig XS, Gelisse P, Crespel A, Genton P. Senile myoclonic epilepsy: delineation of a common condition associated with Alzheimer's disease in Down syndrome. *Seizure* 2010; **19**: 383–9.

Moller JC, Hamer HM, Oertel WH, Rosenow F. Late-onset myoclonic epilepsy in Down's syndrome (LOMEDS). *Seizure* 2001; **10**: 303–6.

Sangani M, Shahid A, Amina S, Koubeissi M. Improvement of myoclonic epilepsy in Down syndrome treated with levetiracetam. *Epileptic Disord* 2010; **12**: 151–4.

Strzelczyk A, Haag A, Raupach H, *et al.* Prospective evaluation of a post-stroke epilepsy risk scale. *J Neurol* 2010; **257**: 1322–6.

Vignoli A, Zambrelli E, Chiesa V, *et al.* Epilepsy in adult patients with Down syndrome: a clinical-video EEG study. *Epileptic Disord* 2011; **13**: 125–32.

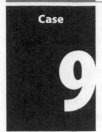

Case

9

When laughing makes the child fall down

Barbara Fiedler and Gerhard Kurlemann

Clinical history

A mother comes with her 10 ¼- year-old daughter to the neuropediatrican. The daughter shows developmental delay. The mother reports on "drop attacks" on laughter in her daughter during the last months.

General history

Birth history was uneventful. In the neonatal period she had hyperbilirubinemia with no necessity of phototherapy. The girl achieved developmental milestones at a normal rate until the age of 3 years. From that time, she lost acquired motor skills and impairment in mental development became more obvious.

Examination

The girl showed severe ataxia, a nearly complete loss of speech, and urinary and stool incontinence. We provoked laughing and the girl presented short episodes of head nods first, then she suddenly lost general tone leading to a collapse with slumping down. She did not lose consciousness.

Special studies

EEG was normal during these episodes. There was no sudden sleep onset. MRI showed a non-specific global brain atrophy. In the ultrasound of the abdomen a slight splenomegaly appeared . On ophthalmological examination no vertical palsy was seen. In the neurometabolic analysis the activity of serum chitotriosidase was markedly elevated.

Follow-up

Moleculargenetic investigations of the Niemann–Pick gene 1 and 2 (NPC1 and NPC2) revealed two mutations in the NPC1 gene. Therapy with miglustat was initiated, unfortunately with no positive effect on the cataplectic episodes.

Diagnosis

Cataplexy. In this case symptomatic cataplexy in Niemann–Pick Disease Type C (NPC disease).

General remarks

Cataplexy is described as a brief episode of bilateral loss of muscle tone brought on by strong emotions such as laughing, exhilaration, or anger. It is a main symptom in narcolepsy. In childhood it is both very rare and often misdiagnosed as epilepsy or non-epileptic collapse. Cataplexy can also show up symptomatically in diseases with CNS affection such as brain tumors, encephalitis, or head trauma, but also in inherited diseases such as Niemann–Pick Disease Type C, Norrie syndrome, Coffin–Lowry syndrome, Prader–Willi syndrome, and Möbius syndrome.

Niemann–Pick Disease Type C is an autosomal recessive disorder due to mutations in the NPC1 or NPC2 gene. It is a neurovisceral atypical lysosomal lipid storage disorder with a heterogeneous clinical presentation. Depending on the age at onset of the first neurological symptoms, there is a subdivision in a perinatal, early infantile, late infantile, juvenile, and an adult form. The main symptoms are neonatal jaundice (hepato-)splenomegaly, delay in motor milestones, respectively, loss of motor skills, speech delay, school problems, psychiatric problems, ataxia, dysarthria, dysphagia, and dementia. The prognosis largely correlates with the age at onset of the neurological symptoms, as earlier is worse. NPC disease is

---

Case Studies in Epilepsy, ed. Hermann Stefan, Elinor Ben-Menachem, Patrick Chauvel and Renzo Guerrini. Published by Cambridge University Press. © Hermann Stefan, Elinor Ben-Menachem, Patrick Chauvel and Renzo Guerrini 2012.

a severe disorder that leads to premature death in most of the cases. Treatment is symptomatically. Miglustat reversibly inhibits the glycosphingolipid synthesis and is therefore able to stabilize and sometimes even to improve the progredient symptoms of NPC disease.

Suggested reading

Chokroverty S. Overview of sleep and sleep disorders. *Ind J Med Res* 2010; **131**: 126–40.

Mayer G. *Narkolepsie. Taschenatlas Spezial.* Georg Thieme Verlag KG, 2006.

Nishino S, Kanbayashi T. Symptomatic narcolepsy, cataplexy and hypersomnia, and their implications in the hypothalamic hypocretin/orexin system. *Sleep Med Rev* 2005; **9**: 269–310.

Patterson MC, Vecchio D, Prady H *et al.* Miglustat for treatment of Niemann–Pick C disease: a randomised controlled study *Lancet Neurol* 2007; **6**: 765–72.

Smit LS, Lammers GJ, Catsman-Berrevoets CE. Cataplexy leading to the diagnosis of Niemann–Pick disease type C. *Pediatr Neurol* 2006; **35**: 82–4.

Vanier MT. Niemann–Pick disease type C. *Orphanet J Rare Dis* 2010; **5**: 16.

Case 10

Epileptic spasms and abnormal neuronal migration

Francesco Mari and Renzo Guerrini

Clinical history

We evaluated a 19-year-old woman with epileptic spasms, moderate cognitive impairment, and subcortical band heterotopia (Fig. 1, DCX gene mutation at c.557G>C: Arg186Pro) and treated her with antiepileptic drugs without success. She manifested prolonged series of epileptic spasms upon awakening, every day. These series lasted up to 1 hour causing repetitive drop attacks. In order to prevent injuries related to falls, the patient spent most of the morning in bed. At age 27 years, we decided to evaluate for a drug-resistant multifocal epilepsy.

General history

Since age 3 years, brief atypical absences had appeared. Since age 12 years, a more coherent picture had emerged, characterized by epileptic spasms in association with focal motor and atypical absence seizures. Several antiepileptic drugs were introduced without any satisfactory response.

Examination

Neurological examination revealed moderate cognitive impairment. Prolonged video–EEG recordings captured several clusters of epileptic spasms upon awakening (Fig. 2).

Image findings

MRI showed subcortical band heterotopia.

Follow-up

At 28 years of age, anterior callosotomy was performed with remarkable reduction of the spasms (Fig. 3) and drop attacks.

Diagnosis

Subcortical band heterotopia, drug-resistant epileptic spasms, moderate cognitive impairment.

General remarks

Epileptic spasms are typically observed in the first year of life as infantile spasms in the context of West syndrome or the infantile spasm syndrome. At this age, their appearance is almost invariably associated with developmental impairment and is often accompanied by hypsarrhythmia on the EEG. The

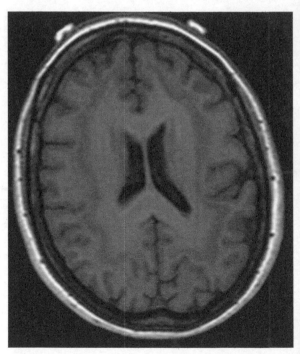

Fig. 1. Axial T1-weighted images showing subcortical band heterotopia.

Case Studies in Epilepsy, ed. Hermann Stefan, Elinor Ben-Menachem, Patrick Chauvel and Renzo Guerrini. Published by Cambridge University Press. © Hermann Stefan, Elinor Ben-Menachem, Patrick Chauvel and Renzo Guerrini 2012.

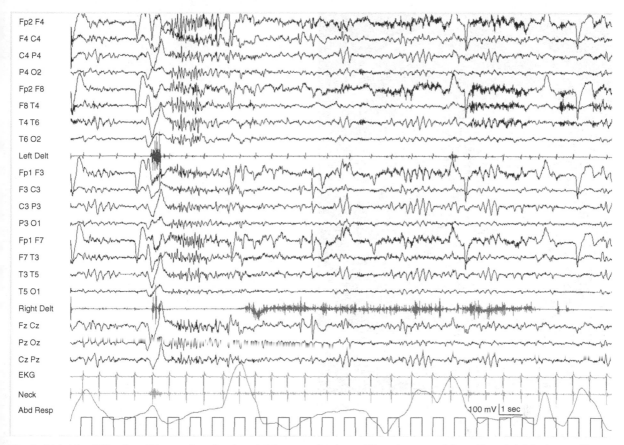

Fig. 2. Ictal video–EEG polygraphic recording showing a brief spasm related to a diffuse slow wave, followed by a brief discharge of low voltage fast rhythm.

occurrence of spasms in older children and adults is rare and is most often associated with a brain malformation and is not accompanied by a hypsarrhythmic EEG.

Special remarks

Subcortical band heterotopia is a neuronal migration disorder characterized by bilateral bands of heterotopic gray matter interposed in the white matter between the cortex and lateral ventricular walls. *LIS1* and *DCX* are the major genes associated with subcortical band heterotopia. As *DCX* is carried on the X chromosome, males with mutations will usually have classical LIS while female patients will have SBH. Epilepsy in patients with SBH can present with a wide range of severity. Symptomatic generalized epilepsy of the Lennox–Gastaut type is particularly frequent, but other types of severe complex epilepsies can be observed. Epileptic spasms with onset beyond

the usual age of infantile spasms should always raise the suspicion of a developmental abnormality of the cerebral cortex.

Future perspectives

Callosotomy should be considered in patients with epileptic drop attacks. There are no criteria to predict the response to this palliative surgical procedure. Patients with similar clinical presentations may either improve remarkably or fail to respond. Repetitive severe drop attacks caused by spasms or tonic seizures are severely disabling for patients who would otherwise walk autonomously. The presence of a diffuse brain malformation should not discourage the procedure, keeping in mind that the ultimate goal of callosotomy is to reduce the drop attacks, their traumatic consequences, and the unavoidable restrictions that the patient experiences as a consequence.

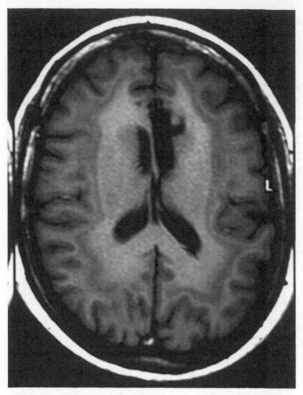

Fig. 3. Post-callosotomy axial T1-weighted image showing the trajectory of neurosurgical approach.

Suggested reading

Camfield P, Camfield C, Lortie A, Darwish H. Infantile spasms in remission may reemerge as intractable epileptic spasms. *Epilepsia* 2003, **44**: 1592–5.

Guerrini R, Parrini E. Neuronal migration disorders. *Neurobiol Dis.* 2010; **38**: 154–66.

Mai R, Tassi L, Cossu M, *et al.* A neuropathological, stereo-EEG, and MRI study of subcortical band heterotopia. *Neurology* 2003; **60**: 1834–8.

Tanriverdi T, Olivier A, Poulin N, Andermann F, Dubeau F. Long-term seizure outcome after corpus callosotomy: a retrospective analysis of 95 patients. *J Neurosurg* 2009; **110**: 332–42.

11

A feeling of gooseflesh

Katrin Hüttemann and Hermann Stefan

Clinical history

A 75-year-old woman was referred to the neurological outpatient department. She had experienced for 6 years already episodes with a taste of mushrooms in her mouth and gooseflesh. Shortly afterwards, she normally started shivering. These episodes occurred in a regular 5-week rhythm with up to 20 episodes per day.

General history

The patient has suffered from a mild depression since the death of her husband 10 years ago. Colon carcinoma was diagnosed about 7 years ago, which led to a hemicolectomy.

Examination

The reflexes of the upper limbs were reduced, paresthesia to 4/8 on both sides. The rest of the medical and neurological examination was normal.

Special studies

Laboratory data were insignificant. The patient was referred with the diagnosis of psychogenic non-epileptic seizures. This diagnosis was particularly considered because of the patient history. To speed up the diagnosis the patient was admitted for a video–EEG monitoring. It was possible to detect five seizures with irregular breathing and repetitive speaking ("mushroom, mushroom, ..."). 15–26 seconds after the clinical symptoms, the EEG showed theta-waves with a high amplitude anterior-temporal on the left side.

Follow-up

After the video–EEG telemetry, a therapy with oxcarbazepine was started. With this medication the patient showed only two seizures in 8 months, but she complained about double vision. Due to this adverse reaction, the treatment was changed to topiramate, which showed a very good improvement of the symptoms with only approximately two very short and mild seizures a month.

Diagnosis

Focal seizures.

General remarks

Psychogenic non-epileptic seizures are involuntary episodes of behavior, movement, or sensation that may mimic epileptic seizures. They are one of the most important differential diagnoses of epilepsy, but this differential diagnosis of epileptic seizures is often very challenging and, due to the different treatment regimens, it is important to find the correct diagnosis.

Video–EEG is the gold standard in the diagnostic work-up to differentiate between seizures of neurologic origin and non-epileptic seizures. This is even more important as some patients with complex partial seizures present with very uncommon symptoms.

It was found that, in about 25% of the patients, the initial diagnosis changed after video–EEG telemetry. In most of the cases these were patients who were initially diagnosed with epileptic seizures. Only a small percentage of the patients with psychogenic non-epileptic seizures also have epilepsy (5%–10%).

Case Studies in Epilepsy, ed. Hermann Stefan, Elinor Ben-Menachem, Patrick Chauvel and Renzo Guerrini. Published by Cambridge University Press. © Hermann Stefan, Elinor Ben-Menachem, Patrick Chauvel and Renzo Guerrini 2012.

Suggested reading

Alsaadi TM, Thieman C, Shatzel A, Rarias S. Video–EEG telemetry can be a crucial tool for neurologists experienced in epilepsy when diagnosing seizure disorders. *Seizure* 2004; **13**: 32–4.

Benbadis SR, Agrawal V, Tatum WO. How many patients with psychogenic nonepileptic seizures also have epilepsy? *Neurology* 2001; **57**: 915–17.

Krebs PP. Psychogenic nonepileptic seizures. *Am*

J Electroneurodiagnostic Technol. 2007; **47**: 20–8.

Reuber, M. Psychogenic nonepileptic seizures: answers and questions. *Epilepsy Behav* 2008; **12**: 622–35.

Case

12

Generalized epilepsy in adolescence as initial manifestation of Lafora disease

Renzo Guerrini and Melania Falchi

Clinical history

A 17-year-old girl from Children's Hospital A. Meyer-University of Florence with a history of drug-resistant generalized epilepsy with absence, myoclonic and tonic–clonic seizures, marked photosensitivity, and cognitive slowing.

The onset of epilepsy occurred at age 12 years with brief absence seizures and photic-induced jerks. A first EEG showed normal background; no neurological signs were present. The clinical and electrographic picture remained unchanged for the following 2 years until a relevant and global worsening occurred.

General history

Parents are first-degree cousins.

Neurological examination

Cerebellar signs (ataxia, dysmetria, and adiadochokinesia), action and spontaneous myoclonus, combined with mental slowness and ideomotor apraxia.

Special studies

Video–EEG recordings showing, since age 15, slowing of background activity with brief absence seizures accompanied by 3 Hz spike and polyspike and wave discharges. Photic-induced myoclonic jerks. Progressive slowing of background activity and evidence of occipital abnormalities in subsequent recordings were noticed.

Evoked potentials (VEPs and SEPs) revealed giant cortical components.

Follow-up

Seizures were drug resistant. Clinically, the cognitive status worsened and generalized and multifocal myoclonus became increasingly severe.

Current treatment: piracetam, valproate, ethosuximide, phenobarbital.

Image findings

Brain MRI was normal.

Diagnosis

Lafora disease (progressive myoclonic epilepsy-2B, EPM2B with a c.205C>G substitution in the malin gene, NHLRC1).

General remarks

The Lafora type progressive myoclonic epilepsy is an autosomal recessive disease with clinical onset in late childhood or adolescence. At onset, the clinical picture is one of rare generalized myoclonic, tonic–clonic, or absence seizures, which tend to become drug resistant with an insidious course. Occipital seizures and photosensitivity have also been reported. Cortical myoclonus and cognitive decline become progressively obvious. The outcome is often fatal within 5–10 years. Lafora disease is genetically heterogeneous (80% of cases exhibit mutations/deletions of the EMP2A laforin gene in 6q24.3; while the less common EPM2B variant is caused by mutations of the NHLRC1 malin gene at 6p22.3. A third locus has been hypothesized. The EEG at the onset shows normal background and is not unlike that of idiopathic generalized epilepsy (Fig. 1). Photosensitivity is usually present. The EEG pattern quickly becomes much more typical: the background activity slows down, the paroxysmal bursts begin to look more like fast spike-wave and polyspike and wave, and focal, particularly occipital anomalies begin to show up. The physiological sleep patterns tend to disappear (Fig. 2). Histologic studies of multiple tissues, including brain,

Case Studies in Epilepsy, ed. Hermann Stefan, Elinor Ben-Menachem, Patrick Chauvel and Renzo Guerrini. Published by Cambridge University Press. © Hermann Stefan, Elinor Ben-Menachem, Patrick Chauvel and Renzo Guerrini 2012.

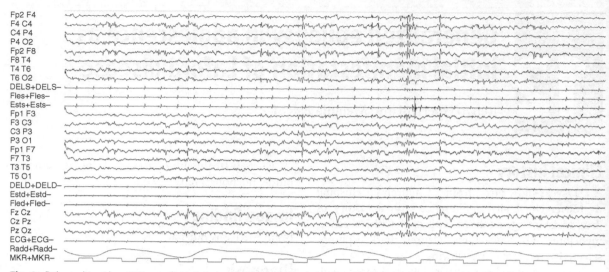

Fig. 1. Polygraphic video–EEG recording during wakefulness. Marked slowing of background activity, multiple spikes, and polyspikes discharges, which are inconstantly related to focal distal myoclonic jerks over the left wrist flexors and extensors (Ests = Left extensors; Estd = Right extensors; Fles = Left flexors; Fled = Right flexors).

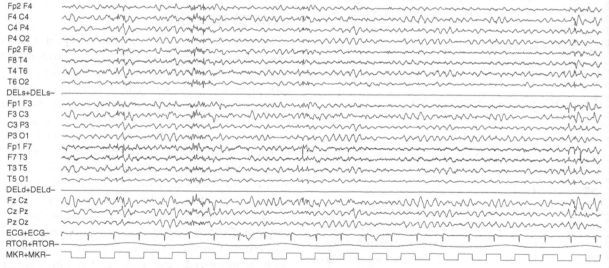

Fig. 2. Polygraphic video–EEG recording during slow wave sleep. Physiological sleep elements are absent. There are brief, diffuse, polyspike discharges.

muscle, liver, and heart show intracellular Lafora bodies, which are dense accumulations of malformed and insoluble glycogen molecules, termed polyglucosans. Lafora bodies are found in myoepithelial cells surrounding axillary apocrine (odoriferous) glands, whereas outside the axilla, Lafora bodies are found in the cells composing the ducts of the eccrine (perspiration) glands. Axillary biopsy has been used for diagnostic purposes for many years. Nowadays molecular genetic testing is often performed directly even before a bioptic study when the clinical suspicion arises.

Special remarks

The progressive electroclinical and cognitive deterioration was not obvious in the first 2 years after seizure onset. As often happens a presumptive diagnosis of

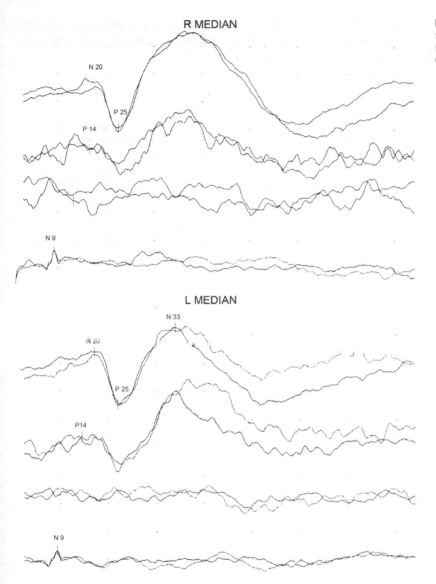

R MEDIAN

L MEDIAN

Fig. 3. Cortical SEP to electrical stimulation of both median nerves at wrist shows a bilaterally enlarged N20-P25-N33 complex (giant potentials).

idiopathic generalized epilepsy was made. However, parental first-degree consanguinity should make one suspicious of the possibility of an autosomal recessive disease. Monitoring EEG activity, especially background EEG, is of special help for orienting the diagnosis. Polygraphic recordings of myoclonic jerks, SEPs and VEPs, are simple and effective tools that support the diagnostic suspicion of progressive myoclonus epilepsy (Fig. 3). Age at onset and rate of progression can direct towards a specific disease. Age at onset in the late school age or early adolescence are typically seen in Lafora disease.

Future perspectives

There is at present no specific treatment for Lafora disease and the only way to alleviate its course is to combine antiepileptic drugs that may reduce seizures and myoclonus. Drugs such as valproate and benzodiazepines are usually preferred. Piracetam has a powerful antimyoclonic effect at very high doses. However, the benefit that can be obtained with antiepileptic and antimyoclonic drugs is time limited. New perspectives are emerging from a better understanding of the genetic basis of the disease. Genotype and haplotype analyses indicate that reduced activity of the protein targeting glycogen (PTG), which is coded by the PPP1R3C gene, may be associated with a slow progression of the disease through decreased capacity to induce glycogen synthesis, making PTG a potential target for pharmacogenetic and therapeutic approaches.

Suggested reading

Delgado-Escueta AV. Advances in Lafora progressive myoclonus. *Curr Neurol Neurosci Rep* 2007; 428–33.

Delgado-Escueta AV, Bourgeois BF. Debate: does genetic information in humans help us treat patients? PRO – genetic information in humans helps us treat patients. CON – genetic information does not help at all. *Epilepsia* 2008; **49**: 13–24.

Guerrero R, Vernia S, Sanz R, *et al*. A PTG variant contributes to a milder phenotype in Lafora disease. *PLoS One* 2011; **6**: e21294.

Lesca G, Boutry-Kryza N, de Toffol B, *et al*. Novel mutations in EPM2A and NHLRC1 widen the spectrum of Lafora disease. *Epilepsia* 2010; **51**: 1691–8.

Monaghan TS, Delanty N. Lafora disease: epidemiology, pathophysiology and management. *CNS Drugs* 2010; 549–61.

Singh S, Ganesh S. Lafora progressive myoclonus epilepsy: a meta-analysis of reported mutations in the first decade following the discovery of the EPM2A and NHLRC1 genes. *Hum Mutat*. 2009; **30**: 715–23.

Turnbull J, DePaoli-Roach AA, Zhao X, *et al*. PTG depletion removes Lafora bodies and rescues the fatal epilepsy of Lafora disease. *PLoS Genet* 2011; 7.

13

Epilepsy with a right temporal hyperintense lesion in MRI

Frank Kerling and Hermann Stefan

Clinical history

A 33-year-old patient developed epigastric auras, tonic–clonic and complex partial seizures 6 months before admission to our epilepsy center.

Examination

On neurological examination, he had no pathological findings except gaze-evoked nystagmus. The neuropsychological evaluation pointed to a slightly lower verbal memory.

Special studies

Initial MRI revealed normal findings, but cerebrospinal fluid (CSF) analysis detected discrete lymphocytosis (15/µl) and positive oligoclonal bands as well as slightly elevated protein levels (552 mg/l). Three months later, a second MRI showed a small hyperintense lesion within the right amygdala without any contrast enhancement, but with a volume increase (Fig. 1). CSF findings were unchanged and screening for neurotropic viruses (herpes simplex, varicella-zoster, cytomegalovirus, Epstein–Barr, measles, spring summer meningo-encephalitis, human herpes-6), or borrelia did not reveal any specific infection. Because of the pharmacoresistant seizures, the patient was admitted to our presurgical evaluation program. During video–EEG monitoring, we were able to record 17 complex partial seizures with oral and manual automatisms as well as tachycardia and a right temporomesial seizure pattern. Intracarotid amobarbital testing showed intact hippocampal functions of both hemispheres and speech dominance was lateralized to the left hemisphere.

Follow-up

Because of the structural MRI lesion of unknown etiology and pharmacoresistance a selective amygdalohippocampectomy was performed. The histology of a surgical specimen, including hippocampus and amygdala, revealed prominent microglial nodules as well as infiltrating T-lymphocytes compatible with a diagnosis of limbic encephalitis (LE). Tumor staging was initiated and an embryonal carcinoma of the right testis was detected. Anti-MA2-antibody titers were greatly increased with a level of 1:25 600. Orchidectomy and respective chemotherapy regimens with platinex, etoposide and bleomycine were performed.

The latest follow-up visit was performed 50 months after epilepsy surgery showing the patient still seizure free with the exception of one withdrawal seizure in the first year, when the patient accidentally forgot his medication. Postoperative verbal and figural memory functions were still normal. The anti-MA2 antibody titers dropped below detection limits after treatment of the tumor.

Diagnosis

Symptomatic epilepsy and paraneoplastic limbic encephalitis.

General remarks

The following diagnostic criteria were previously defined for LE: (i) a compatible clinical picture (personality changes, irritability, depression, seizures, memory loss, dementia); (ii) an interval of <4 years between the development of neurological symptoms and tumor diagnosis; (iii) exclusion of other neuro-oncological complications; and

Case Studies in Epilepsy, ed. Hermann Stefan, Elinor Ben-Menachem, Patrick Chauvel and Renzo Guerrini. Published by Cambridge University Press. © Hermann Stefan, Elinor Ben-Menachem, Patrick Chauvel and Renzo Guerrini 2012.

(a)

(b)

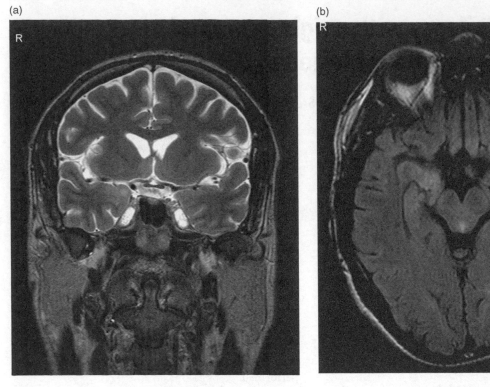

Fig. 1. Coronal T2-weighted image (left) and axial FLAIR TSE image (right): hyperintense signal changes were visible within the amygdala of the right hemisphere, no significant signal increase in left amydgala.

(iv) at least one of the following features: CSF with inflammatory changes but negative cytology; MRI demonstrating temporal lobe abnormalities; EEG showing epileptic activity in the temporal lobes. When LE is diagnosed, there is a need to initiate onconeural antibody detection. Although there are cases of non-paraneoplastic LE, e.g., LE with voltage gated potassium channel (VGKC)-antibodies, tumor screening should always be performed. Positive onconeural antibodies may lead to a specific tumor entity. Anti-Ma2-antibodies (also called anti-Ta-antibodies), for example, are often detected in patients with testicular tumors or lung cancer. Chest X-ray, abdominal ultrasound, urological, and gynecological examinations should be included, but whole body FDG-PET seems to remain the gold standard for tumor screening.

Special remarks

The clinical course and the diagnostic findings in our case were not typical with respect to the LE criteria. Whereas LE is characterized by clinical symptoms such as temporal lobe seizures, memory deficits, and psychiatric symptoms, our patient did not develop memory decline nor psychiatric symptoms. Histological diagnoses of LE and the positive Ma2-antibodies lead to embryonal carcinoma.

Suggested reading

Bien CG, Urbach H, Schramm J, *et al.* Limbic encephalitis as a precipitating event in adult-onset temporal lobe epilepsy. *Neurology* 2007; **69**: 1236–44.

Dalmau J, Graus F, Villarejo A, *et al.* Clinical analysis of anti-Ma2-associated encephalitis. *Brain* 2004; **127**: 1831–44.

Gultekin SH, Rosenfeld MR, Voltz R, *et al.* Paraneoplastic limbic encephalitis: neurological symptoms, immunological findings and tumour association in 50 patients. *Brain* 2000; **123**: 1481–94.

Hoffmann LA, Jarius S, Pellkofer HL, *et al.* Anti-Ma and anti-Ta associated paraneoplastic neurological syndromes: 22 newly diagnosed patients and review of previous cases. *J Neurol Neurosurg Psychiatry* 2008; **79**: 767–73.

Vedeler CA, Antoine JC, Giometto B, *et al.* Management of paraneoplastic neurological syndromes: report of an EFNS Task Force. *Eur J Neurol* 2006; **13**: 682–90.

Vincent A, Buckley C, Schott JM, *et al.* Potassium channel antibody-associated encephalopathy: a potentially immunotherapy-responsive form of limbic encephalitis. *Brain* 2004; **127**: 701–12.

Case 14

Epileptic falling seizures associated with seizure-induced cardiac asystole in drug-resistant temporal lobe epilepsy

Guido Rubboli, Stefano Meletti, Marco Giulioni,
Anna Federica Marliani, Yerma Bartolini, Stefano Forlivesi,
Elena Gardella, and Roberto Michelucci

Clinical history

A 52-year-old gentleman with positive family history for epilepsy. At 1 year of age he suffered from prolonged febrile seizures. At 29 years, he started to present brief episodes of loss of contact, staring and psychomotor arrest, paleness, oro-alimentary and right-hand gestural automatisms; the episodes occurred usually once or twice per month. At 49 years, the episodes increased in frequency and about 50% of them started to be complicated by abrupt and sudden falls to the ground. Despite several antiepileptic treatments, his seizures were never completely controlled. The patient was admitted to undergo long-term video–EEG monitoring for presurgical evaluation.

General history

Arterial hypertension; duodenal ulcer; chronic HVB hepatitis; deep venous thrombosis with pulmonary embolism; thrombophilia (heterozygous factor V Leiden mutation).

Examination

Unremarkable. Right-handed (Oldfield score: +1).

Brain MRI

Right mesial temporal sclerosis (Fig. 1).

Interictal EEG

Sporadic theta activities occasionally associated with spikes during sleep in the right temporal leads.

Long-term video–EEG monitoring

Three stereotyped seizures were recorded during a 10-day computerized video–EEG monitoring. All of them occurred while the patient was sitting, and displayed stereotyped electroclinical features: the clinical onset was characterized by psychomotor arrest, oscillations of the trunk, and then backward fall in two seizures, frontward in the third episode; then oro-alimentary and right-hand automatisms were observed. A very brief postictal state followed. Ictal EEG showed a brief flattening in the right fronto-temporal leads, followed by a rhythmic theta-delta discharge with phase reversal in F8-T4; then delta activity mainly confined to the right temporal leads appeared. The EKG lead showed periods of asystole whose durations ranged from 5 to 8 seconds, associated with the right temporal rhythmic theta activity (Fig. 2), then the heart rate progressively resumed to baseline. The fall of the patient occurred few seconds after the end of the asystole, when the heart rate was starting to recover.

Cardiologic evaluation

Cardiologic examination, echocardiography, continuous heart rate/blood pressure monitoring were unremarkable. During head-up tilt test, a 7-second asystole occurred, consistent with neuromediated syncope.

Follow-up

The patient underwent right antero-mesial temporal lobe resection. Six years after surgery the patient is

Case Studies in Epilepsy, ed. Hermann Stefan, Elinor Ben-Menachem, Patrick Chauvel and Renzo Guerrini. Published by Cambridge University Press. © Hermann Stefan, Elinor Ben-Menachem, Patrick Chauvel and Renzo Guerrini 2012.

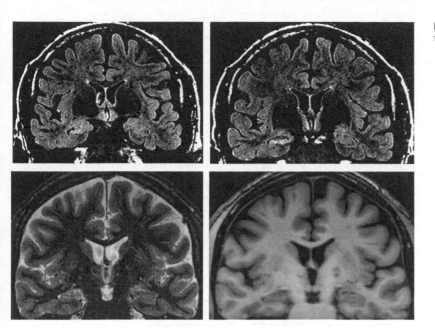

Fig. 1. Brain MRI showing right mesial temporal sclerosis.

seizure free; no more episodes of abrupt falling to the ground occurred.

Diagnosis

Epileptic falling seizures associated with seizure-induced cardiac asystole in drug-resistant temporal lobe epilepsy.

General remarks

Appearance of epileptic falling seizures (EFS) during the evolution of a focal epilepsy is usually considered an ominous sign indicating worsening of the epileptic condition (Lipinski, 1977; Pazzaglia *et al.*, 1985). The pathophysiological mechanisms of EFS are not fully elucidated yet: involvement of bitemporal structures as well as origin from frontal regions with subsequent bilateral spread have been suggested (Ethelberg, 1950; Delgado-Escueta *et al.*, 1982; Tassinari *et al.*, 1997; Tinuper *et al.*, 1998). The observation in the interictal EEG of secondary bilateral synchrony supports the involvement of bilateral cerebral structures, possibly resulting from secondary epileptogenesis. Among the physiopathogenetic mechanisms underlying EFS, the possible role of cardiac arrhythmias associated with ictal EEG discharges, such as ictal bradycardia or cardiac asystole, are usually considered rare phenomena, although

several recent reports have demonstrated the occurrence of marked bradycardia and, eventually, asystole, during focal epileptic seizures (Tinuper *et al.*, 2001; Rocamora *et al.*, 2003; Carvalho *et al.*, 2004; Altenmuller *et al.*, 2004; Rubboli *et al.*, 2008).

Special remarks

In our patient, video–EEG monitoring showed that the ictal epileptic discharges in the right temporal lobe were associated with asystole that caused the abrupt fall to the ground, then typical clinical manifestations of antero-mesial temporal lobe seizures followed. From the EEG point of view, in our patient asystole and the related falls differed from previous EEG documentation of syncopal attacks because of the absence of high amplitude delta activity, maximal anteriorly; commonly interpreted as a sign of cerebral hypoperfusion (Brenner, 1997); indeed, the ictal discharge persisted throughout the bradycardic and asystolic period.

Occurrence of ictal bradycardia/asystole might be underestimated. In fact, our case illustrates that differentiation between seizure-induced asystole and syncope sometimes cannot be made on strict clinical grounds and might be anamnestically difficult. Syncope and epileptic seizures are manifested by "identical symptomatologic features: loss of consciousness,

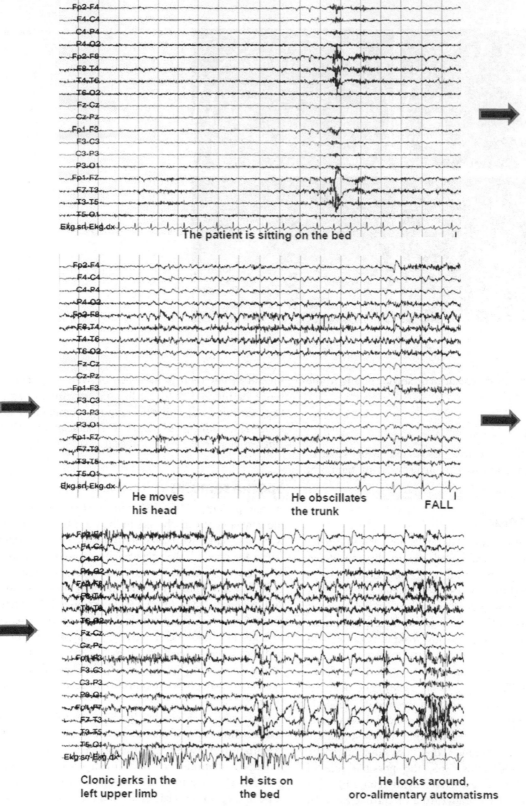

Fig. 2. Ictal EEG showing a theta–delta rhythmic discharge in the right temporal leads with phase reversal in F8-T4, associated with a 7-second asystolia (middle panel). The fall of the patient occurs, after a few oscillations of the trunk, when the cardiac rhythm starts to recover. Interval between vertical bars: 1 second.

dilatation of the pupils, tonic convulsions, clonic jerks, abundant salivation, passing of urine and feces, and postictal fatigue sometimes accompanied by vomiting and occasionally requiring the patient to seek repose in sleep" (Gastaut, 1974).

Recognition of severe bradycardia or cardiac asystole associated with epileptic seizures can be of paramount importance in the management of epileptic patients. Indeed, cardiac arrhythmias are usually considered to play a role in sudden death in epilepsy (SUDEP), and implantation of a cardiac pacemaker is considered in patients with drug-resistant focal seizures associated with ictal bradycardia or asystole. In addition, evidence of ictal bradyarrhythmias may warn against the administration of potentially arrhythmogenic antiepileptic drugs (such as, for instance, carbamazepine). Our case report suggests that the appearance of EFS in the evolution of a focal epilepsy should be properly investigated by polygraphic (EEG–EKG) recording of the ictal events.

Suggested reading

Altenmuller DM, Zehender M, Schulze-Bonhage A. High-grade atrioventricular block triggered by spontaneous and stimulation-induced epileptic activity in the left temporal lobe. *Epilepsia* 2004; **45**: 1640–4.

Brenner P. Electroencephalography in syncope. *J Clin Neurophysiol* 1997; **14**: 197–209.

Carvalho KS, Salanova V, Markand ON. Cardiac asystole during temporal lobe seizure. *Seizure* 2004; **13**: 595–9.

Delgado-Escueta AV, Enrile-Bacsal F, Treiman DM, *et al.* Complex partial seizures on closed-circuit television and EEG: a study of 691 attacks in 79 patients. *Ann Neurol* 1982; **11**: 292–300.

Ethelberg S. Symptomatic "cataplexy" or chalastic fits in cortical lesions of the frontal lobe. *Brain* 1950; **53**: 499–511.

Gastaut H. Syncopes: generalized anoxic cerebral seizures. In PJ Vinken, GW Bruyn, eds. *Handbook of Clinical Neurology*, vol **15**. Amsterdam: The Netherlands, 1974: 815–35.

Lipinski C. Epilepsies with astatic seizures of late onset. *Epilepsia* 1977; **18**: 13–19.

Pazzaglia P, D'Alessandro R, Ambrosetto G, Lugaresi E. Drop attacks: an ominous change in the evolution of partial epilepsy. *Neurology* 1985; **35**: 1725–30.

Rocamora R, Kurthen M, Lickfett L, von Oertzen J, Elger CE. Cardiac asystole in epilepsy: clinical and neurophysiologic features. *Epilepsia* 2003; **44**: 179–85.

Rubboli G, Bisulli F, Michelucci R, *et al.* Sudden falls due to seizure-induced cardiac asystole in drug-resistant focal epilepsy. *Neurology* 2008; **70**: 1933–5.

Tassinari CA, Michelucci R, Shigematsu H, Seino M. Atonic and falling seizures. In J Engel, T Pedley, eds, *Epilepsy: A Comprehensive Textbook*. Philadelphia: Lippincott-Raven Publishers, 1997: 605–616.

Tinuper P, Cerullo A, Marini C, *et al.* Epileptic drop attacks in partial epilepsy: clinical features, evolution and prognosis. *JNNP* 1998; **64**: 231–7.

Tinuper P, Bisulli F, Cerullo A, *et al.* Ictal bradycardia in partial epileptic seizures: autonomic investigation in three cases and literature review. *Brain* 2001; **124**: 2361–71.

Seizures, dementia, and stroke?

15

Björn Holnberg and Elinor Ben-Menachem

This man was born in 1923 and is today 87 years old. He has been healthy for most of his life and has a treated hypertension. He had generalized tonic–clonic seizures, one in 1993, one in 1998, and one in 2001. He was started on valproate in 2001 after the last seizure. His CT scans in 1999 and 2001 were both normal. He was seen for the first time at our clinic for a follow-up in 2004. Since then he has been feeling fine and there have been no other seizure episodes.

In November 2008 he presented with right-sided partial status epilepticus emanating from the temporal lobe. He was put into the intensive care unit and treated with fosphenytoin, propofol, and an increased dose of valproate, after which the status stopped after 2 hours. A new CT scan showed slight atrophy with changes in the white matter, spread throughout the two hemispheres.

After coming out of status epilepticus, he had a left-sided weakness, which was interpreted as an ischemic stroke. He was confused, classed as demented, sleepy, incontinent, and had a left-sided action tremor. One year earlier, this man was able to take care of himself and live an active life. Now plans were being made to put him in a home for demented patients.

The EEG in November 2008 did not show epileptic activity but a lack of alpha rhythm and a general 7 Hz background. This was interpreted as general encephalopathy and therefore a CSF study was done, which showed an increased NFL (neurofilament light protein) of 2020 ng/l (normal value is <750 ng/l) and increased tau of 700 ng/l (normal value is <400 ng/l).

The diagnoses considered at that were: stroke, dementia, Jakob–Creutzfeldt, normal pressure hydrocephalus, Parkinson, and valproate encephalopathy.

Although serum ammonia levels were not increased (22 µmol/l), the decision to stop valproate and switch to carbamazepine was made as a first step. He had been treated with valproate for 7 years, so it was felt that this was a long shot but worth a try. Down-titration of valproate was started in November 2008.

After valproate had been completely eliminated, but not before the last dose, this patient had become more awake and started to be interested in training his arms and legs. By January 2009 he could stand and started to walk. His dementia-like condition disappeared entirely. By January 2009 he was back to his usual social activities and had a better memory.

In 2011 levetiracetam was added to his carbamazepine monotherapy, since he still had an occasional seizure. He can now walk with the help of a walker, is continent and not demented. At the last CT scan in May 2009, the atrophy and the white matter changes were described as before. The EEG in August 2009 had normalized with an increase in background activity now at 10 Hz. There are, however, now some sporadic interictal spikes seen on the right side around the temporal lobe.

Lessons learned

Valproate encephalopathy should be considered in older patients who suddenly become demented or confused for no other apparent reason. Even if the ammonia level is not increased, encephalopathy can occur after several years of treatment. The good news is that valproate-induced encephalopathy will disappear when valproate is withdrawn completely. Since there are now many other AEDs to choose from, valproate should be used with caution in older

Case Studies in Epilepsy, ed. Hermann Stefan, Elinor Ben-Menachem, Patrick Chauvel and Renzo Guerrini. Published by Cambridge University Press. © Hermann Stefan, Elinor Ben-Menachem, Patrick Chauvel and Renzo Guerrini 2012.

patients. There has been discussion about whether carnitine supplementation could be effective in countering valproate encephalopathy even when not induced by an increase in ammonia. In one study the dosage of valproate negatively correlated with total and free carnitine levels.

There is a high prevalence of dementia associated with hypocarnitine, but controlled randomized studies would be needed to better elucidate the relationship between valproate-induced encephalopathy and prophylactic treatment with carnitine.

Suggested reading

Cuturic M, Abramson RK, Moran RR, Hardin JW, Hall AV. Clinical correlates of low serum carnitine levels in hospitalized psychiatric patients. *Wld J Biol Psychiatry* 2010 Jun 29. [Epub ahead of print]

Lheureux PE, Hantson P. Carnitine in the treatment of valproic acid-induced toxicity. *Clin Toxicol (Phila)*. 2009; 47: 101–11.

Comorbidity in epilepsy – dual pathology resulting in simple focal, complex focal, and tonic–clonic seizures

Thilo Hammen and Hermann Stefan

Clinical history

A 34-year-old man came to our epilepsy center for preoperative diagnostics. Since the age of 14 years he has suffered from simple focal seizures demonstrating unclear foreshadowing, hard to explain for the patient. Duration: several seconds, frequency: twice per month. In addition, he suffers from complex partial seizures involved with gazing, oral automatism, no reaction to speech, and pausing. Duration: 10–40 seconds, frequency: twice per month. The patient told us that 15 years ago tonic–clonic seizures occurred additionally.

Examination

The right-handed patient suffers from decline of verbal memory, furthermore, regular findings in clinical neurological examination.

Neurological examination

Normal.

Special studies

Video–EEG monitoring

Interictal: theta-focus and spiking in the frontotemporal right region.

Ictal: eight complex focal seizures were recorded with clinical features described above. The EEG pattern started with decrement of amplitude and high frequency activity frontotemporal right; in the course of monitoring development of rhythmic theta activity with high amplitude in the described region.

Cranial MRI

Hippocampal sclerosis in the right temporal lobe with atrophy in coronal inversion recovery slices (Fig. 1) and hyperintensity of hippocampal structures in T2-weighted images (Fig. 2). In addition, signal alteration in the entorhinal cortex, gyrus parahippocampalis and occipitotemporalis in the right hemisphere, suspicious for cortical dysplasia.

Cognitive testing

Cognitive testing demonstrated a specific impairment of verbal memory displaying a mesiotemporal lesion. Because lesions were found in the right mesial temporal lobe in MRI a WADA test was recommended.

WADA test

The WADA test showed a left hemispheric speech localization and a good global functioning of the left hippocampal structures. The right hippocampal structures demonstrated a significant dysfunction. The results of the WADA test demonstrated that, from neuropsychological side of view, there was no contraindication for a right temporal resection.

Routine laboratory tests: unremarkable.

Follow-up

The patient suffered from intractable temporal lobe epilepsy. The findings of the special studies mentioned above were discussed in the interdisciplinary epilepsy conference. Surgery was recommended.

Case Studies in Epilepsy, ed. Hermann Stefan, Elinor Ben-Menachem, Patrick Chauvel and Renzo Guerrini. Published by Cambridge University Press. © Hermann Stefan, Elinor Ben-Menachem, Patrick Chauvel and Renzo Guerrini 2012.

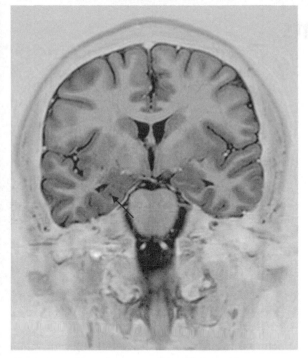

Fig. 1. Coronal inversion recovery of temporomesial structures.

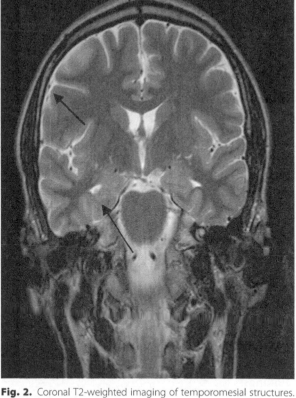

Fig. 2. Coronal T2-weighted imaging of temporomesial structures.

Diagnosis

Symptomatic epilepsy with simple focal, complex focal, and tonic–clonic seizures.

Dual pathology with hippocampal sclerosis and cortical dysplasia in the entorhinal cortex, gyrus parahippocampalis and gyrus occipitotemporalis in the right temporal lobe.

The common physiopathology is still not clearly understood. The epileptogenesis of the lesions has to be determined by electrophysiological investigations (EEG, MEG).

General remarks

Dual pathology in epilepsy is defined as the association of two potentially epileptogenic lesions, which involve hippocampal (sclerosis, neuronal loss) and extrahippocampal (temporal or extratemporal) regions. As in our case, cortical dysplasias are most commonly associated with hippocampal sclerosis. In most cases the lesions are in one hemisphere; only rarely are the lesions located in different hemispheres.

Special remarks

Surgical strategy is determined by the location of both lesions and their relative role in seizure generation. Reported surgical results suggest that simultaneous resection of mesial temporal structures along with the extrahippocampal lesion should be performed. Studies over the last 20 years show that seizure freedom for at least 1 year in 66%–100% of patients with dual pathology is achievable.

Suggested reading

Rougier A. Dual pathology, *Neurochirurgie* 2008; **54**: 382–7.

Spencer S, Huh L. Outcomes of epilepsy surgery in adults and children, *Lancet Neurol* 2008; **7**: 525–37.

17

Minor motor events

Christian Tilz

Clinical history

A 67-year-old female patient introduced herself in our neurological ambulance (Krankenhaus Barmherzige Brüder, Linz) with symptoms of sleep disturbance and extreme tiredness during the day for the past 5 years. Under the diagnosis of "restless-leg syndrome" she was treated unsuccessfully with ropinirole.

General history

Atrial fibrillation.

Examination

Neurologic evaluation suggested no pathological findings.

Special studies

A polysomnography (PSG) performed in our sleep laboratory (Somnomedics Somnoscreen, Germany) revealed short stereotype events several times per minute during non-REM sleep in the night with flexion of the arms and the legs with a mean duration of 2 seconds and a highly reduced sleeping time. Simultaneous two-channel-EEG (C3/C4) recording during PSG captured event-related poly-spikewave complexes.

There was no pathologic finding in a standard scalp EEG, but in a sleep-deprived EEG a bifrontal theta-slowing was shown. In a long-term EEG recording a seizure-onset pattern on F4 was recorded.

A cranial MRT according to the protocol of the ILAE was without pathologic finding.

Follow-up

After treatment with gabapentin (900 mg daily dose), the patient was nearly seizure free. After increasing the dose to 1500 mg, complete seizure freedom was achieved.

Image findings (Figs. 1, 2, 3)

Diagnosis

Nocturnal frontal lobe epilepsy (NFLE) with minor motor events (MME).

General remarks

Nocturnal seizures are not seldom encountered. They belong to a group of difficult-to-diagnose seizures, not only because they are normally unperceived, but also because of the diversity of nocturnal sleep-related events. These seizures often occur during the switch phase from REM sleep to non-REM sleep, i.e., the seizure activity could probably be provoked during REM sleep and could propagate to non-REM sleep. Long-term video–EEG monitoring can help to differentiate between nocturnal epileptic seizures and non-epileptic seizures.

Special remarks

MMEs are epileptic seizures occurring during non-REM sleep and are one type of nocturnal frontal lobe epilepsy. They are characterized by periodic stereotypic movements of limb and trunk for 2–4 seconds, often with arousal. Therefore, in such patients sleep efficiency can be greatly reduced

Case Studies in Epilepsy, ed. Hermann Stefan, Elinor Ben-Menachem, Patrick Chauvel and Renzo Guerrini. Published by Cambridge University Press. © Hermann Stefan, Elinor Ben-Menachem, Patrick Chauvel and Renzo Guerrini 2012.

(a)

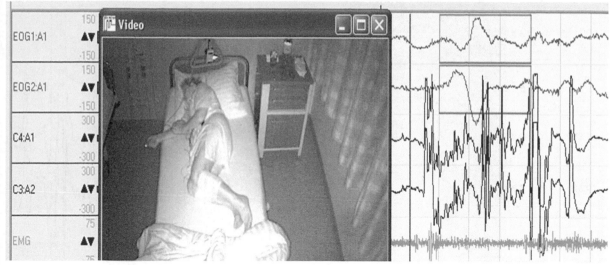

Fig. 1(a). Flexions of the limbs with polyspikewave activity in EEG during polysomnography.

(b)

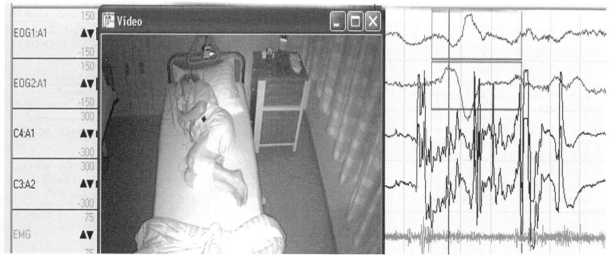

Fig. 1(b). Frontal slowing during sleep EEG.

and excessive day-time sleepiness often occurs. Patients with NFLE may have MME as the only seizure type. Sometimes in the same patient, MME can be observed together with other major motor events such as dystonic movements, which was formerly called nocturnal paroxysmal dystonia and might last 20–30 seconds.

In our case, the semiology of the patient had been misinterpreted for several years as restless-leg syndrome and had been inappropriately treated. The combination of PSG and a long-term EEG helped to make a correct diagnosis and an optimal therapy was launched, which not only led to a freedom from seizures, but also to the disappearance of sleep disturbance and day-time fatigue.

Future perspective

Combination of PSG with simultaneous video–EEG monitoring will be necessary for clarification of those unclear nocturnal events and also for an optimal clinical intervention.

(c)

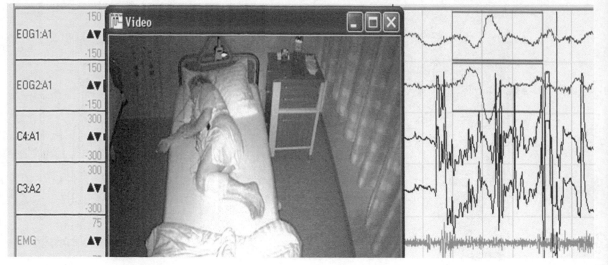

Fig. 1(c). Flexions of the limbs with polyspikewave activity in EEG during polysomnography.

Suggested reading

Gardella E, Rubboli G, Tassarini CA. Ictal grasping: prevalence and characteristics in seizures with different semiology. *Epilepsia* 2006; 47: 59–63.

Nobili L, Sartori I, Terzaghi M, *et al.* Relationship of epileptic discharges to arousal instability and periodic leg movements in a case of nocturnal frontal lobe epilepsy: a stereo-EEG study, *Sleep* 2006; 29: 701–4.

Parriano L, Smerieri A, Spaggiari MC, Terzano MG. Cyclic alternating pattern (CAP) and epilepsy during sleep: how a physiological rhythm modulates a pathological event. *Clin Neurophysiol* 2001; 111: 39–46.

Terzaghi M, Sartori I, Mai R, *et al.* Sleep-related minor-motor-events in nocturnal frontal lobe epilepsy. *Epilepsia* 2007; 48: 335–41.

Tezaghi M, Sartori I, Mai R. Coupling of minor motor events and epileptiform discharges with arousal fluctuations in NFLE. *Epilepsia* 2008; 49: 670–6.

Terzano MG, Monge-Strauss MF, Mikol F, *et al.* Cyclic alternating pattern as a provocative factor in nocturnal paroxysmal dystonia. *Epilepsia* 1997; 38: 1015–25.

Wieser HG. Temporal lobe epilepsy, sleep and arousal: stereo-EEG findings. *Epilepsy Res* 1991; 2: 97–119.

Epilepsy in the ring chromosome 20

18

Anca Pasnicu, Patrick Chauvel, and Arnaud Biraben

Clinical history

Here is the case of a 12 years 7 months old right-handed girl who was referred for epilepsy surgery evaluation because of a very active recent epilepsy resulting in therapeutic escalade.

The epilepsy started 7 months before admission to our unit. There were several types of seizures. During wakefulness she had seizures with progressive hypertonia with axial anterior flexion and lateral abduction of the superior limbs starting usually on the left side, then symmetrical. She was unresponsive and had mydriasis. After a dozen seconds the hypertonia became fragmented, sometimes with associated synchronous rhythmic vocalization. Then the patient seemed to try to catch the objects around her with both hands. The facial expression also changed and she seemed terrified. Finally, she relaxed and had gestural and oro-alimentary automatisms with impaired contact. These seizures lasted up to 1 minute. She began to respond verbally soon after the end of the seizure, without focal neurological deficit, but with an intense fatigue. The patient did not report any prodromal symptoms, but was sometimes aware that she had had a seizure. Some of these seizures were preceded by long periods (more than 20 minutes) when she seemed slowed down in her movements, sometimes even prostrated and totally unresponsive, or walking around without purpose, talking and responding inappropriately. She was partially amnesic of these episodes. During sleep she had hypertonic episodes that seemed sometimes to start more abruptly than during wakefulness. Other times, before the nocturnal seizures, she woke up, sat down on the side of the bed, her face seeming scared, then she had a sudden anterior flexion of the trunk for 10–20 seconds, followed by the usual slow recovery.

The antiepileptic treatment was started rapidly after the beginning of the epilepsy: valproate was tried first. Because the seizures persisted, the bitherapy valproate–oxcarbazepine was tried, then oxcarbazepine–carbamazepine, oxcarbazepine–carbamazepine–levetiracetam. The current treatment is oxcarbazepine–carbamazepine–clonazepam. Despite this treatment, the seizures became more and more frequent. She has currently one to two seizures every afternoon, three to four seizures during the evening and one dozen during the night. Confusional episodes preceding the seizures are reported almost every evening. Sometimes they end with a hypertonic seizure that may repeat over a few minutes without recovery of normal consciousness.

The school results were average before the beginning of the epilepsy. Since then, she hasn't been to school.

General history

She is the fourth of five children of a non-consanguineous family, her four brothers being in good health. Her development during early childhood is reported as normal. There is no significant family and personal history.

Examination

Physical and neurological examination are normal.

Neuropsychological assessment

Neuropsychological assessment was attempted 2 months after the beginning of the epilepsy, but it was difficult to perform because of an important fatigue and frequent seizures. The neuropsychological profile seems quite harmonious.

Case Studies in Epilepsy, ed. Hermann Stefan, Elinor Ben-Menachem, Patrick Chauvel and Renzo Guerrini. Published by Cambridge University Press. © Hermann Stefan, Elinor Ben-Menachem, Patrick Chauvel and Renzo Guerrini 2012.

Special studies

Video–EEG recordings show a mild slowing of the background activity at 8 Hz on the posterior leads, with poor organization and poor attenuation by the eyes opening, and this is stable from the beginning of the epilepsy. Paroxysmal abnormalities are multifocal and increase during sleep (Fig. 1). Many seizures have been recorded: they begin during wakefulness or during non-REM sleep. They are more or less clinically similar (see above), but electrically they can begin by right perisylvian slow spikes that accelerate into a diffuse discharge with right anterior predominance, or by an initial rhythmic bilateral anterior spike discharge that slows down irregularly. During the second part of the seizure there is a rhythmic diffuse slow spike-and-wave complex activity lasting about 1 minute. Therefore, these hypertonic seizures are not stereotyped and are difficult to classify. Some of these seizures are preceded by obnubilation episodes that last several dozens of minutes and correspond to activities with sudden onset and end of diffuse bilateral frontal irregular rhythmic high-voltage theta waves mixed with spikes (Fig. 2). These activities last between several seconds and several minutes, repeat during dozens of minutes and often end with a hypertonic seizure. The interictal and ictal data suggest a large multifocal bilateral cerebral involvement. The clinical and electrophysiological features of these seizures associated with the obnubilation states that sometimes precede them as well as the interictal patterns are characteristic of the epilepsy related to the ring chromosome 20 [r(20)] syndrome.

Image findings

The cerebral MRI is normal.

Diagnosis

Diagnosis of the epilepsy related to a mosaicism of r (20) chromosome was confirmed by the genetic examination performed on 70 cells and 25 mitoses: the ring of the chromosome 20 (Fig. 3) was present in 44% of the analyzed mitoses: her chromosomal

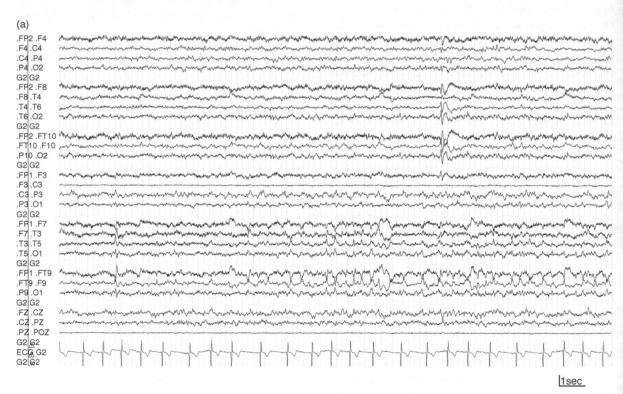

(a)

1sec

Fig. 1. Interictal bilateral multifocal paroxystic abnormalities during wake **(a)** and during sleep **(b)**: slow temporo-perisylvian spike-and-wave complexes; synchronous and asynchronous bilateral perisylvian-temporal spikes, isolated, in bursts or discharges (longitudinal bipolar montage; calibration signal: 1 sec, 100 μV/cm, low filter 0,530 Hz, high filter 120 Hz; FP10, FP9: anterior basal temporal; P10, P9: posterior basal temporal).

(b)

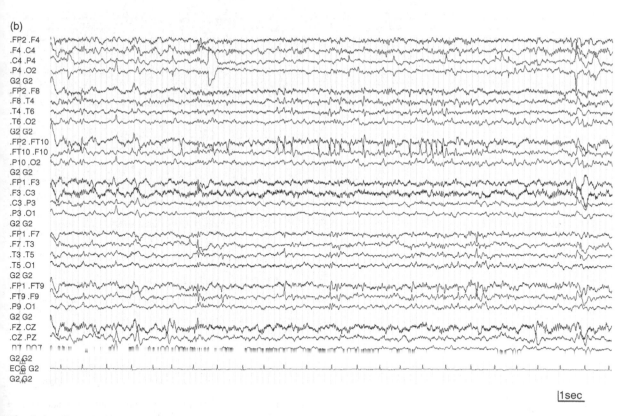

|1sec

Fig. 1. (*cont.*)

formula is mos 46, XX, r(20) [11]/46, XX [14]. The karyotype of both parents is normal.

Follow-up

Carbamazepine and clonazepam were progressively stopped and phenytoin was added to the oxcarbazepine. Since the adjunction of the phenytoin, all the hypertonic seizures have disappeared but the patient still has frequent obnubilation episodes.

General remarks

Epilepsy in r(20) syndrome is a rare chromosomal disorder, which has a peculiar electroclinical pattern (Inoue *et al.*, 1997; Canevini *et al.*, 1998). Epilepsy is the main clinical feature of this chromosomal syndrome. Epilepsy begins most often during childhood (range 1 day–14 years). The r(20) syndrome is more difficult to diagnose in very young children because they have shorter complex partial seizures and their

epilepsy lacks the more characteristic seizures (Ville *et al.*, 2006). The latest develop after the age of three. The most characteristic features are prolonged confusional episodes that last from several minutes to 1 hour (real absence status), associated with seizures with fear linked to terrifying visual hallucinations, loss of contact, motor, and oro-alimentary automatisms. Long-lasting absence status is frequent, often daily. Other seizures include hypertonic seizures especially during sleep and other focal complex seizures. Background EEG activity may be normal or slow. Obnubilation episodes correspond to long-lasting high-voltage frontal or diffuse irregular rhythmic theta activities mixed with occasional spikes. The epilepsy is drug resistant, but exceptionally it may miss. There is significant phenotypic variability concerning neuropsychological and dysmorphic features. Often, there are acquired variable developmental and behavioral disturbances that accentuate after epilepsy onset (Vignoli *et al.*, 2009). Dysmorphic features are

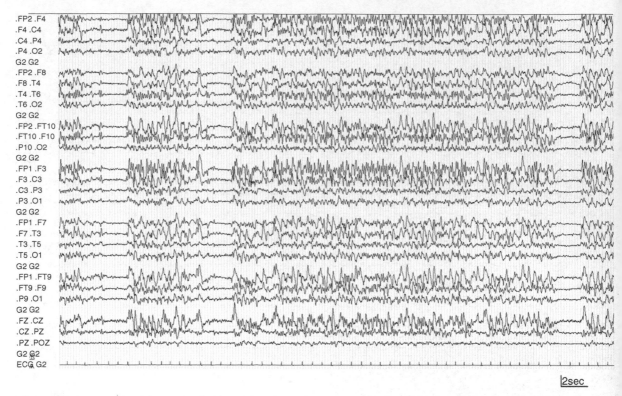

Fig. 2. EEG during an obnubilation episode: bilateral frontal irregular rhythmic theta waves of high-voltage mixed with spikes (longitudinal biporal montage; calibration signal: 2 sec, 250 μV/cm, low filter 0.530 Hz, high filter 120 Hz; FP10, FP9, P10, P9: see **Fig. 1**).

Fig. 3. Karyotype of the patient, r(20).

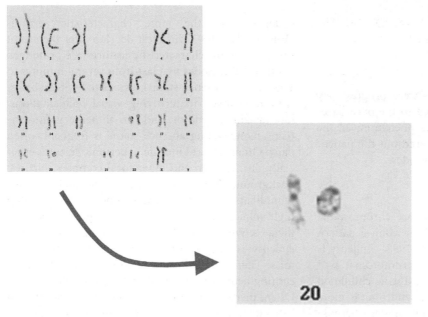

rare and unspecific (microcephaly, wide forehead, hypoplastic toenails). Whether early onset and severity of the neurological features are linked to the percentage of cells exhibiting the r(20) chromosome also remains controversial (Augustijn *et al.*, 2001; Nishiwaki *et al.* 2005; Ville *et al.*, 2006; Giardino *et al.*, 2010), but could be linked to the size of the telomeric deletion leading to the ring formation.

Special remarks

The electroclinical features of seizures in the patient that we report, and particularly the obnubilation states with characteristic EEG pattern strongly suggested r(20) syndrome, which was confirmed by genetics. This patient has very active drug-resistant large multifocal epilepsy; classical surgical treatment is not an option. Generally, the best results are obtained with antiepileptic drugs used for generalized epilepsy such as valproate and lamotrigine, but the epilepsy of our patient was well improved by the phenytoin–oxcarbazepine bitherapy. Besides medical treatment, other therapeutic options may be discussed, such as

vagal nerve stimulation or deep stimulation methods, which are still experimental.

Future perspectives

The pathogenic epilepsy mechanism is still unknown. The genetic investigations conducted by Giardino *et al.* (2010) suggest that the phenotypic and neurologic features of the r(20) syndrome may be underlined by an epigenetic mechanism perturbing the genes close to telomeric regions, rather than by the deletion of genes located at the distal 20p and 20q regions. Aside from that, several studies have confirmed the involvement of dopamine neurotransmission in seizure activity of the r(20) syndrome and other refractory epilepsies (Starr, 1996; Bouilleret *et al.*, 2005). Moreover, for some authors the prolonged confusional states could result from an abnormality of the endogenous seizure-terminating mechanisms (Biraben *et al.*, 2004). These pathogenic hypotheses will necessarily lead to exploration of new therapeutics of the epilepsy in the r(20) syndrome.

Suggested reading

Augustijn PB, Parra J, Wouters CH, *et al.* Ring chromosome 20 epilepsy in children: electroclinical features. *Neurology* 2001; **57**: 1108–11.

Biraben A, Semah F, Ribeiro MJ, *et al.* PET evidence for a role of the basal ganglia in patienhts with ring chromosome 20 epilepsy. *Neurology* 2004; **63**: 73–7.

Bouilleret V, Semah F, Biraben A, *et al.* Involvement of the basal ganglia in refractory epilepsy: an [18]Fluoro-L-Dopa PET study using 2 methods of analysis. *J Nucl Med* 2005; **46**: 540–7.

Canevini MP, Sgro V, Zuffardi O, *et al.* Chromosome 20 ring: a chromosomal disorder associated with a particular electroclinical pattern. *Epilepsia* 1998; **39**: 942–51.

Giardino D, Vignoli A, Ballarati L, *et al.* Genetic investigations in 8 patients affected by ring 20 chromosome syndrome. *BMC Med Genet* 2010; **11**: 146.

Inoue Y, Fujiwara T, Matsuda K, *et al.* Ring chromosome 20 and nonconvulsive status epilepticus: a new epileptic syndrome. *Brain* 1997; **120**: 939–53.

Nishiwaki T, Hirano M, Kumazawa M, Ueno S. Mosaicism and phenotype in ring chromosome 20 syndrome. *Acta Neurol Scand* 2005; **111**: 205–8.

Starr MS. The role of dopamine in epilepsy. *Synapse* 1996; 159–94.

Vignoli A, Canevini MP, Darra F, *et al.* Ring chromosome 20 syndrome: a link between epilepsy onset and neuropsychological impairment in three children. *Epilepsia* 2009; **50**: 2420–7.

Ville D, Kaminska A, Bahi-Buisson N, *et al.* Early pattern of EEG in ring chromosome 20 syndrome. *Epilepsia* 2006; **47**: 543–9.

Case

19

A late diagnosis of mesial temporal lobe epilepsy

Anca Pasnicu, Patrick Chauvel, Claire Haegelen, and Arnaud Biraben

Clinical history

A 30-year-old patient was referred for presurgical evaluation of an active and handicapping drug-resistant partial epilepsy.

At the age of 5 he was operated on for appendicular peritonitis.

Immediately after, he began to experience episodes of abdominal pain, sometimes followed by restlessness. These episodes lasted less than 5 minutes, and were considered as functional and digestive in origin. No other diagnosis was made during his childhood. These episodes frequently recurred and, only after several marked episodes with impaired contact at the age of 17, were additional neurological examinations performed. Epilepsy was therefore diagnosed and antiepileptic drug treatment was started, then adapted, but never successful in controlling the seizures.

The patient can now report that the symptomatology of his seizures has been unchanged since his childhood. He is experiencing about ten seizures per month, often occurring in clusters over a few days. During these "bad days" he claims that he has a permanent background of epigastric pain. The onset of a fit is signalled to him by a brisk increase of epigastric pain intensity, associated with a feeling of anxiety. Sometimes he can warn verbally of the seizure onset. Then he loses contact and the family reports that he becomes pale, has oro-alimentary automatisms and eructation, and then is briefly agitated. He doesn't fall, and doesn't drop the objects that he may have in his hands at the time of seizures. The seizures usually last 2 to 3 minutes. He doesn't have postictal language deficit nor long-lasting amnesia or disorientation. He is always aware of having presented a seizure. He has never had status epilepticus or secondary generalized seizures.

General history

He has no personal or family significant pathological history.

Examination

He is the only left-handed member of his family. His general and physical examinations are normal.

Special studies

Posterior background EEG activity was normal. There were frequent anterior right temporal sharp waves (Fig. 1) and sometimes rhythmic delta activities. There were also rare anterior and basal right temporal spikes when the patient had seizures. During video–EEG monitoring it became clear that the abdominal pain background of the "bad days" was actually made up of repeated episodes of epigastric pain of 1-minute duration that repeated over several hours. The EEG appeared generally quite normal during these sensations, but sometimes there was only asymmetric fading of the background activity over the right temporal region. Seven seizures with loss of contact were recorded during a "bad day."

They are stereotyped. The patient had a tachycardia as an inaugural clinical sign. A few seconds later, he signalled a non-ascending epigastric pain, then had oro-alimentary automatisms, eructation, and left upper limb dystonia. There was a late and incomplete loss of contact; then got agitated and presented imitation behavior. He didn't have any language disturbance at the onset or after the seizures, but during their second half he might tell sentences out of context. There was no postictal visual field defect.

Ictal EEG was stereotyped from seizure to seizure (Fig. 2). Video–EEG electroclinical data were

Case Studies in Epilepsy, ed. Hermann Stefan, Elinor Ben-Menachem, Patrick Chauvel and Renzo Guerrini. Published by Cambridge University Press. © Hermann Stefan, Elinor Ben-Menachem, Patrick Chauvel and Renzo Guerrini 2012.

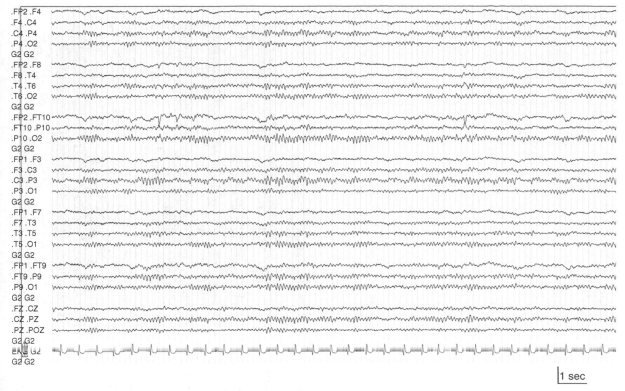

Fig. 1. Interictal EEG: normal posterior background activity, right anterior temporal sharp waves (longitudinal montage; FT10, FT9 anterior basal temporal; P10,P9 posterior basal temporal; calibration signal: 1 sec, 100 μV/cm, low filter 0.530 Hz, high filter 120 Hz).

conformed to the diagnosis of mesial temporal seizure within a non-dominant hemisphere for language.

Neuropsychological assessment

Total IQ: 85; verbal IQ: 88; performance IQ: 85. Language and the memory assessment were normal, without any asymmetry for the latter. He made several confusions in face recognition and had a tendency to make rotations in construction tests. So, there was a weak global development and a mild right temporal dysfunction.

Image findings

He had right hippocampal sclerosis at MRI examination (Fig. 3). The interictal and the ictal SPECT (Fig. 4) pointed to anterior and medial right temporal lobe involvement. There was also ictal hyperperfusion of the lateral right temporal region and of the right insular cortex.

Diagnosis

Electroclinical features, morphological and functional imaging data, as well as neuropsychological assessment were in favor of the diagnosis of right medial temporal epilepsy. These data also allowed establishing that the right hemisphere was non-dominant for language, despite left-handed manual lateralization. This epilepsy was drug-resistant and very handicapping. Therefore, a right anterior and medial temporal lobectomy including the temporal pole, the hippocampus and the amygdala, and the anterior part of the superior and middle temporal gyri was proposed as a surgical treatment.

Follow-up

He was operated on at the age of 30, soon after video–EEG monitoring. Pathological analysis confirmed hippocampal sclerosis. Now he is 37 years old and has been seizure free since surgery (Engel class 1a) and treatment-free for 2 years.

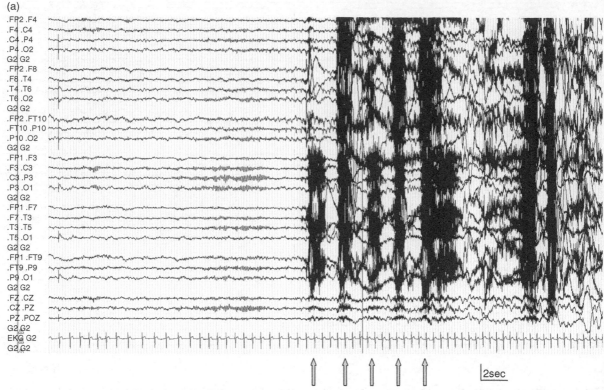

Fig. 2. Ictal EEG (a): right large temporal discharge of rhythmic slow spikes, maximal on the right anterior temporal region. The arrow indicates the artifacts of the early oro-alimentary automatisms that persist until the end of the seizure (longitudinal montage; FT10, FT9, P10, P9 see **Fig. 1**; calibration signal: 2 sec, 100 µV/cm, low filter 0.530 Hz, high filter 120 Hz).
Ictal EEG continued (b): the right temporal discharge spreads progressively on the posterior right areas (longitudinal montage; FT10, FT9, P10, P9 see **Fig. 1**; calibration signal: 2 sec, 150 µV/cm, low filter 1000 Hz, high filter 30 Hz).
Ictal EEG continued (c): late moderate right posterior perysylvian and mild contralateral spread (longitudinal montage; FT10, FT9, P10, P9 see **Fig. 1**; calibration signal: 2 sec, 150 µV/cm, low filter 1000 Hz, high filter 30 Hz).
Ictal EEG end (d): slow propagation to the frontal regions at the end of the seizure (longitudinal montage; FT10, FT9, P10, P9 see **Fig. 1**; calibration signal: 2 sec, 150 µV/cm, low filter 0.530 Hz, high filter 120 Hz).

At neuropsychological assessment 6 months after surgery, there was a mild decline in global memory aptitudes without lateralization, although the patient had no complaint concerning his memory performance in everyday life.

General remarks on clinical diagnosis of temporal seizures

Temporal lobe epilepsy is better known than other focal epilepsies, partly because this is the most common epilepsy referred to epilepsy surgery centers. Temporal seizures are therefore well documented by non-invasive and deep video–EEG recordings. Using intracerebral stimulations and recordings, Penfield and Jasper (1954), and then Bancaud (1987) and Bancaud *et al.*, (1965) described the symptoms and signs of the various temporal seizures and their localizing value. They also showed that, in order to establish individual anatomo-electroclinical correlation, all the clinical signs and symptoms of the seizures should be analyzed as a coherent sequence integrated with physiology and anatomy knowledge. Many authors studied the temporal epilepsies (see Suggested reading). The main diagnostic features of mesial temporal epilepsy with hippocampal sclerosis may be summarized as follows: genetic predisposition to febrile convulsion; a precipitating factor often before the age of 5, the most often a complex febrile convulsion; epilepsy onset generally between 4 and 16 years old, with a variable latency interval after the precipitating factor; characteristic aura with progressive unpleasant ascending epigastric sensation, anxiety, experiential phenomena (dreamy state, déjà-vu, paroxysmal reminiscences),

(b)

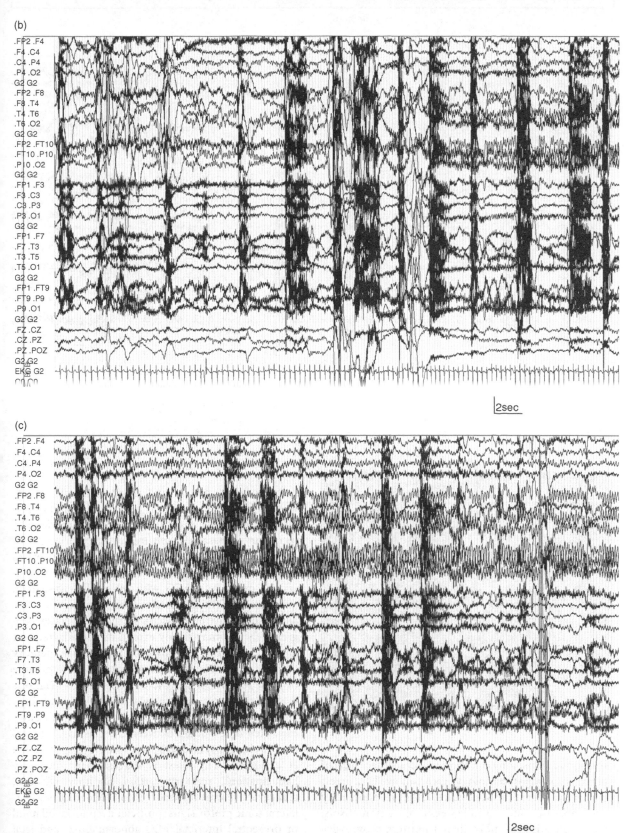

2sec

(c)

2sec

Fig. 2. (cont.)

(d)

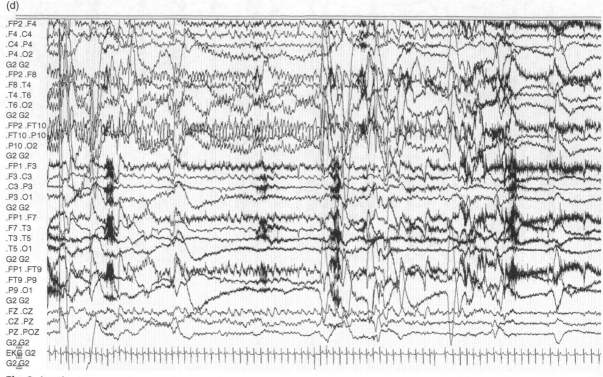

Fig. 2. (cont.)

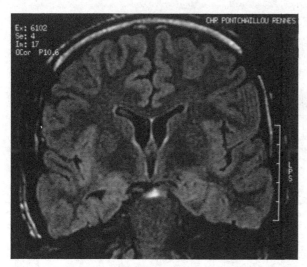

Fig. 3. MRI: right temporal mesial sclerosis.

autonomic signs; long duration (dozens of seconds) of subjective sympatomatology; then followed by arrest of activity, alteration of contact, early oro-alimentary automatisms, and simple gestural automatisms; seizure duration of more than 1 minute; progressive

recovery with amnesic and mood postictal disturbance, and language postictal deficit if the seizure originates from the dominant hemisphere; exceptionally, secondary generalized seizures; usually drug resistance; interictal EEG anterior temporal sharp waves that may be bilateral but predominant on the side of seizure onset; ictal EEG with bilateral or ipsilateral attenuation of the interictal activity followed by lateralized theta rhythmic discharge that accelerates progressively and may slowly extend its spread; frequent episodic memory impairment, and verbal memory deficit if epilepsy is in the dominant hemisphere. None of these features is specific or necessary to diagnosis that is made on congruence of clinical and EEG arguments (Wieser, 2004). Ictal electroclinical findings can often differentiate between the classical "purely" temporal epilepsy and temporal "plus" epilepsy (Barba *et al.*, 2007). The latest is suggested by: gustatory hallucinations, rotatory vertigo, auditory illusions, contraversive eyes or head version, piloerection, ipsilateral tonic motor signs, postictal dysphoria; bilateral or precentral interictal EEG abnormalities, and ictal

(a)

(b)

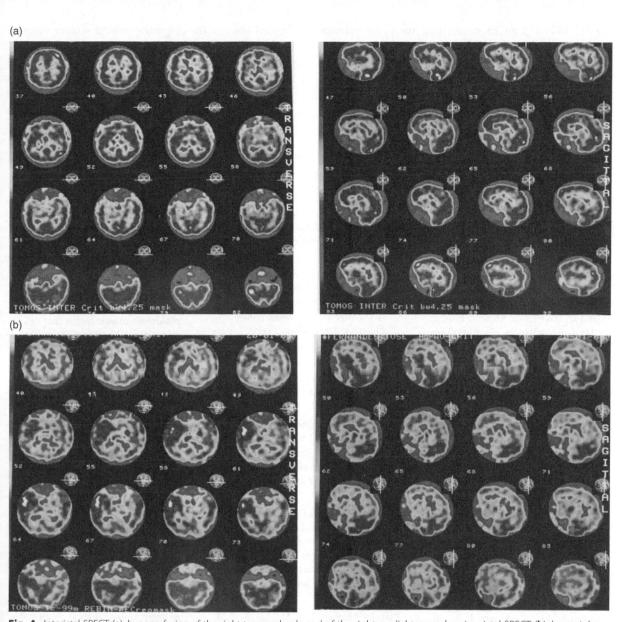

Fig. 4. Interictal SPECT (**a**): hypoperfusion of the right temporal pole and of the right medial temporal region. Ictal SPECT (**b**): large right temporal hyperperfusion extended to the lateral temporal regions and to the left insula (axial left, sagittal right). See color plate section.

anterior frontal, temporo-parietal, and precentral involvement. In order to improve the surgical prognosis of the temporal epilepsies, it is obviously very important to identify these features that suggest involvement of extratemporal areas.

Special remarks

The delay of the epilepsy diagnosis is noteworthy in this case. This was due to the abdominal pain being the main initial and isolated subjective sign at the onset of each seizure that, in addition, started just after abdominal digestive surgery. In this patient the epileptic origin of the abdominal pain episodes was therefore recognized after more than 10 years delay, when loss of contact was noted during longer seizures. In epileptic patients the unpleasant abdominal ascending aura is found more often in temporal (52% of patients) than in extratemporal epilepsies (Henkel *et al.*, 2002). And it is more frequent in mesial (64%) than in neocortical temporal seizures (39%). However, the abdominal aura is neither specific nor always present. Hence it should not be considered in isolation. If an abdominal aura integrates in a coherent clinical sequence, together with autonomic signs and simple automatisms, the probability of temporal epilepsy is important. Isnard *et al.* (2004) also reported ascending epigastric sensation during the direct stimulation of the anterior insular cortex and emphasized the role of the insula in pain sensation.

Exacerbation of the epigastric pain at seizure onset in our patient might therefore be related to fast ictal spread to the insula. Ictal SPECT showed extended right temporal hyperperfusion. Nevertheless, in this patient the strong concordance between all the non-invasive clinical and paraclinical findings converged to an origin of the epilepsy in medial temporal structures, and invasive EEG recordings weren't considered necessary or justified. The diagnosis was finally confirmed by favorable long-term surgical outcome.

Suggested reading

Bancaud J. [Clinical semiology of the seizures of temporal origin]. *Rev Neurol* 1987; **143**: 392–400.

Bancaud J, Talairach J, Bonis A, *et al.* [*The Stereo-Electroencephalography in Epilepsy*] 1965; Paris: Mason.

Barba C, Barbati G, Minotti L, *et al.* Ictal clinical and scalp-EEG findings differentiating temporal lobe epilepsies from temporal 'plus' epilepsies. *Brain* 2007; **130**: 1957–67.

Biraben A, Taussig D. [Seizures of the temporal lobe] *Jalon P. Epilepsies. Volume 2. [Epileptic Seizures, Syndromes and Risk Factors]. Wolters Kluwer*, 2007, 31–43.

Fish DR, Gloor P, Quesney FL, *et al.* Clinical responses to electrical brain stimulation of the temporal and frontal lobes in patients with epilepsy. Pathophysiological implications. *Brain* 1993; **116**: 397–414.

French JA, Williamson PD, Thadani VM, *et al.* Characteristics of medial temporal lobe epilepsy: I. Results of history and physical examination. *Ann. Neurol* 1993; **34**: 774–80.

Henkel A, Noachtar S, Pfänder M, Lüders H. The localizing value of the abdominal aura and its evolution. *Neurology* 2002; **58**: 271–6.

Isnard J, Guénot M, Sindou M, Mauguière F. Clinical manifestation of insular lobe seizures: a stereo-electroencephalographic study. *Epilepsia* 2004; **45**: 1079–90.

Maillard L, Vignal JP, Gavaret M, *et al.* Semiologic and electrophysiologic correlations in temporal lobe seizure subtypes. *Epilepsia* 2004; **45**: 1590–9.

McIntosh A, Kalnins R, Mitchell L, *et al.* Temporal lobectomy: long-term seizure outcome, late recurrence and risks for seizure recurrence. *Brain* 2004; **127**: 2018–30.

Munari C, Bancaud J, Bonis A, *et al.* [Role of amygdala in the occurrence of oro-alimetary signs during epileptic seizures in man (author's transl)]. *Rev Electroencephalogr Neurophysiol Clin* 1979; **9**: 236–40.

Pfänder M, Arnold S, Henkel A, *et al.* Clinical features and EEG findings differentiating mésial from neocortical temporal lobe epilepsy. *Epileptic Disord* 2002; **4**: 289–95.

Penfield W, Jasper HH. *Epilepsy and the Functional Anatomy of the Human Brain*, 1954; Boston: Little Brown.

Semah F, Picot MC, Adam C, *et al.* Is the underlying cause of epilepsy a major prognostic factor for recurrence? *Neurology* 1998; **51**: 1256–62.

Van Buren J. The abdominal aura. A study of abdominal sensation occurring in epilepsy and produced by depth stimulation. *EEG Clin Neurophysiol* 1963; **15**: 1–19.

Wieser H, ILAE Commision of neurosurgery of epilepsy. ILAE Commission Report. Mesial temporal lobe epilepsy with hippocampal sclerosis. *Epilepsia* 2004; **45**: 695–714.

Williamson P, French JA, Thadani V, *et al.* Characteristics of medial temporal lobe epilepsy: II. Interictal and ictal scalp electroencephalography, neuropsychological testing, neuroimaging, surgical results and pathology. *Ann Neurol* 1993; **34**: 781–7.

Case

20

Experiential phenomena in temporal lobe epilepsy

Anca Pasnicu, Yves Denoyer, Arnaud Biraben, and Patrick Chauvel

Clinical history

An 11-year-old boy presented with drug-resistant partial epilepsy. He was referred for presurgical evaluation. The patient is right-handed; his mother is the single left-handed member of the family.

The first seizure occurred at the age of 18 months: the patient was found by his mother abnormally somnolent and hypotonic, he had vomited. Her mother saw afterwards intermittent saccadic movements of the boy's limbs, possibly with a right predominance. No fever was noted at the time of this first seizure and no other cause was identified. No treatment was started at that time.

The second seizure with motor signs occurred at the age of nine. Initially, the boy warned that he wasn't feeling well, then he lost consciousness. His mother reported that he was again having saccadic movements of limbs and of mouth. The emergency medical unit noticed a left deviation of the eyes, right hemiparesis, and coma. Intravenous benzodiazepines and phenytoin were administered with complete recovery during transfer to the hospital.

Diagnosis of epilepsy was made at the age of 9, after the second seizure with motor signs. Only retrospectively his family reported that, since the age of 8, he presented, every 2 to 3 months, stereotyped brief episodes. At that time they were described as an unpleasant anguish memory of a scene similar to what happened at school in the past. The patient was perfectly capable of distinguishing between the voluntary recall of this memory and these episodes of distressing feeling of immersion in a vivid dream with image and sound. The real scene had happened almost 1 year before: he had once been put back in line by his teacher at the entrance to classes after he jumped forward a few places to trifle with his classmates. When these episodes occurred, he was able to signal them to his parents, telling them "I am thinking." There was no associated sign. The onset and the end of these episodes were sudden. According to the patient, they were lasting for 10 to 20 seconds. Since the age of 10 he hadn't had another paroxysmal reminiscence, but only the initial unpleasant feeling of anguish and a diffuse headache of sudden onset. Nevertheless, he was communicating them in the same way, by telling his family "I am thinking." Now he also reports that, after this initial symptom, he has a kind of internal shiver, difficulty to respond verbally, and also brief difficulty to understand if someone talks to him during the seizures. The current seizures last 20 to 30 seconds and are generally without loss of contact. Now his family notices the speech arrest during seizures. They also note the arrest of on-going activities and that there is word retrieval defect lasting a few minutes after the end of the seizures, but he does not seem to have long-lasting difficulties in understanding.

The seizures persist despite four antiepileptic drugs in mono- and polytherapy. At admission, the patient medication was carbamazepine and oxcarbazepine in high doses. The seizures occur every 2 or 3 days, when the patient is awake. The patient hasn't presented any secondary generalized seizures since the treatment was started, but had two episodes of partial status epilepticus triggered by treatment changes.

General history

No significant personal and family history, normal development during early childhood, and normal school results.

Case Studies in Epilepsy, ed. Hermann Stefan, Elinor Ben-Menachem, Patrick Chauvel and Renzo Guerrini. Published by Cambridge University Press. © Hermann Stefan, Elinor Ben-Menachem, Patrick Chauvel and Renzo Guerrini 2012.

Examination

General and neurological examinations are normal.

Special studies

At 18 months the EEG showed occasional diffuse left temporal slow waves. After the second seizure with motor signs, the EEG showed in addition a few left temporo-parietal slow spikes. One EEG performed later on was normal. We performed prolonged video–EEG monitoring. Background activity was normal during wakefulness as well as sleep organization. Left anterior temporal paroxysmal spiking and slow abnormalities (Fig. 1) sometimes became very abundant, at other times they were rare by intervals of minutes or hours. Sometimes they were organized in slow rhythmic discharges with progressive onset and increase in amplitude during several dozens of seconds. Anterior left temporal spikes became very abundant close to the seizures. There was no contralateral abnormality. Several

seizures were recorded: the boy warned suddenly "here I am thinking" as he usually had done ever since childhood. He retrospectively reported that he now signals the diffuse headache and the unpleasant usual initial feeling, without any more experiential hallucinations. Then he follows with the eyes what is happening around him, but he doesn't respond verbally. There are only mild autonomic signs associated. There is no loss of contact, and the seizures last 1 to 2 minutes. Before the end of the seizures and postictally, he briefly has difficulty in understanding simple verbal orders, then presents briefly a jargonaphasia, but the more prolonged (2 minutes) deficit is the word retrieval defect (anomia). He also has a brief right facial paresis. When he can respond verbally, he is well oriented and doesn't have significant postictal amnesia nor postictal visual field defect. At clinical onset of the seizure, the interictal spikes disappear and are followed several seconds afterwards by an anterior left temporal discharge of rapid rhythmic spikes (Fig. 2).

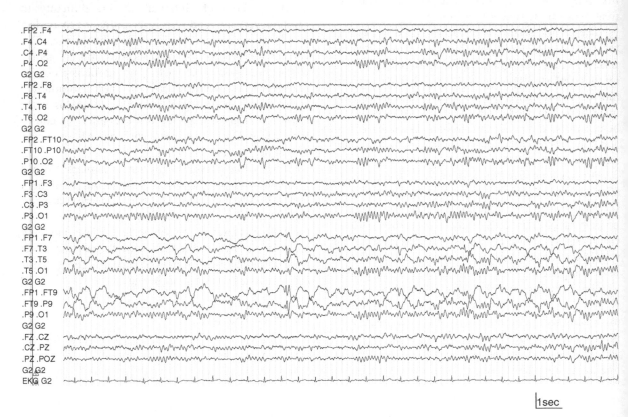

Fig. 1. Interictal EEG: normal posterior background activity. Slow waves mixed with slow spike-wave complexes located on the left anterior temporal derivations (longitudinal montage; FT10, FT9 anterior basal temporal; P10, P9 posterior basal temporal; calibration signal: 1 sec, 150 μV/cm, low filter 0.530 Hz, high filter 120 Hz).

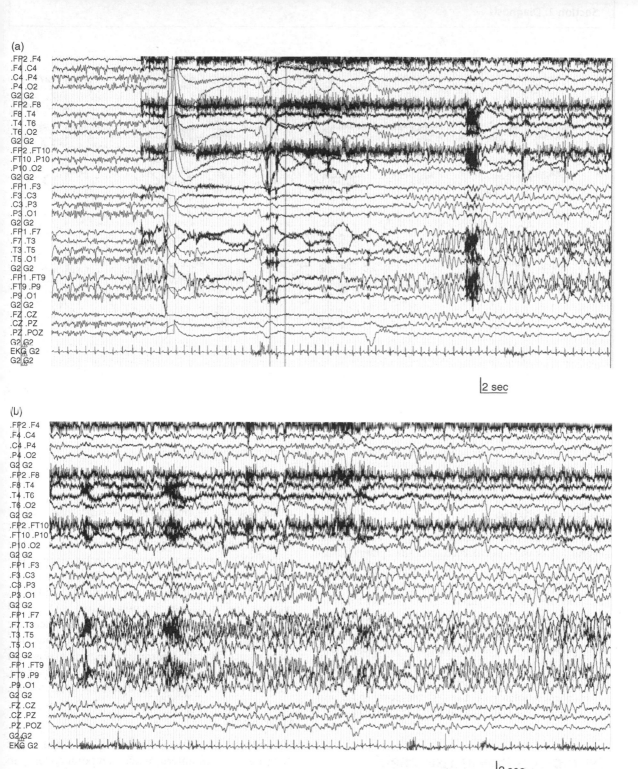

(a)

2 sec

(b)

2 sec

Fig. 2. Ictal EEG (a): at clinical onset, the interictal left anterior spikes disappear, then there is an anterior left temporal discharge of rhythmic spikes, followed rapidly by a brief rhythmic slow delta activity in the left superior and basal posterior temporal derivations (longitudinal montage; FT10, FT9, P10, P9: see Fig. 1; calibration signal: 2 sec, 150 μV/cm, low filter 0.530 Hz, high filter 120 Hz).

Ictal EEG continued (b): the left temporal discharge alternatively accelerates and slows down, and progressively diffuses mildly on the entire left temporal lobe, then on the left frontal region and the right temporal derivations (longitudinal montage; FT10, FT9, P10, P9: see Fig. 1; calibration signal: 2 sec, 150 μV/cm, low filter 0,530 Hz, high filter 120 Hz).

(c)

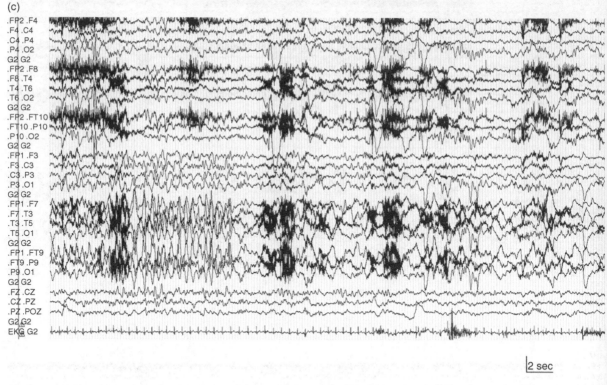

2 sec

Fig. 2. (*cont.*) Ictal EEG end (c): prolonged left temporal post-ictal diffuse slowing (longitudinal montage; FT10, FT9, P10, P9: see Fig. 1; calibration signal: 2 sec, 150 μV/cm, low filter 0.530 Hz, high filter 120 Hz).

Image findings

The cranial CT performed at 18 months was normal. Several MRIs were performed after the epilepsy diagnosis (Fig. 3): there was left hippocampal sclerosis associated with a T2 FLAIR hypersignal of the amygdala and the anterior rhinal region. The MRI abnormalities didn't change on consecutive controls.

Interestingly, ictal SPECT showed significant hyperperfusion of the left temporal pole, especially in its medio-basal part, surrounded by a large hypoperfusion, almost hemispheric (Fig. 4).

Hypometabolism of the left temporal pole and mesial region was evident on the PET scan (Fig. 5).

Neuropsychological assessment

Global cognitive development and intellectual aptitudes were assessed by WISC-IV, which showed a harmonious development above the normal range: total IQ: 100; verbal IQ: 110; perceptive reasoning IQ: 99. Language was assessed by NEPSY tests and all the results are globally above normal. The children clinical assessment scales of memory found: general memory quotient (MQ): 123; immediate and late verbal MQ: 106; verbal recognition: 100; immediate visual MQ: 135; late visual MQ: 125; learning quotient: 125. While there are very mild difficulties in reciting and in names learning, visual and spatial aptitudes are very clearly above normal. There are only mild contaminations at the frontal functions' assessment. Overall, neuropsychological assessment is in favor of epilepsy of the dominant hemisphere, but didn't find any clear and significant focal deficits.

Diagnosis

Clinical and paraclinical findings allow diagnosis of drug-resistant left antero-medial temporal epilepsy in the dominant hemisphere.

Follow-up

The patient continues to have weekly seizures despite the fifth antiepileptic bitherapy. Because all the data are

(a)

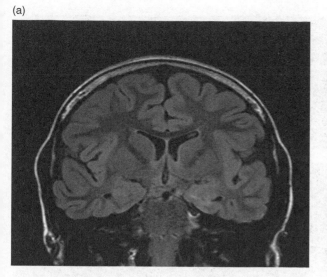

(b)

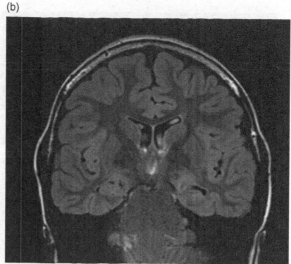

(c)

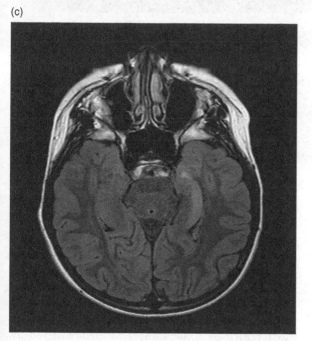

Fig. 3. 3T MRI (a), (b) coronal FLAIR; (c) axial FLAIR: left hippocampal sclerosis; hyper signal of the left amygdala and also of the anterior subhippocampal region extending to the anterior temporal horn of the left lateral ventricle; thickening of the subhippocampal anterior cortex; blurring of the white matter of the left temporal pole.

concordant and his epilepsy is handicapping and drug resistant, we proposed a left temporal cortectomy including the temporal pole, the amygdala, the hippocampus, and the anterior and middle temporal basal cortex. To date, the patient's family has refused a surgical treatment.

General remarks

The exclusively subjective character of experiential seizures at the beginning of the epilepsy history has delayed positive diagnosis. This was all the more difficult to claim as the paroxysmal reminiscence consisted of a scene that really happened in the past. The epilepsy diagnosis was possible only after a more overt seizure associating loss of contact and motor signs occurred, about 1 year after the simple subjective partial seizures started.

Epileptogenic zone localization could be achieved by conjunction of video–EEG and ictal SPECT data. The latter pointed to the anterior medio-basal region of the left temporal lobe.

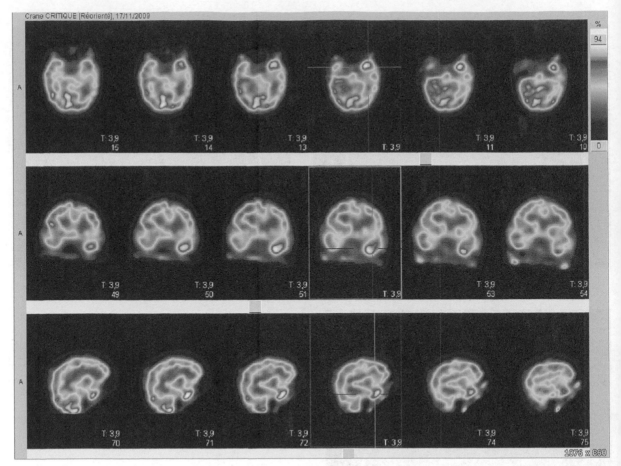

Crane CRITIQUE [Réorienté], 17/11/2009

Fig. 4. Ictal SPECT: significant hyperperfusion of the left temporal pole and left anterior basal temporal region surrounded by a very large ipsilateral hypoperfusion. See color plate section.

MRI features may reflect dysplasia lesion of the anterior rhinal cortex and amygdala associated with left hippocampal sclerosis. This hypothesis is also supported by the electrophysiological interictal frequent anterior temporal spikes and the ictal discharge of rapid spikes, while hippocampal sclerosis alone is generally responsible for sharp theta waves in bursts or discharges and the spikes are rarer (Pfänder *et al.*, 2002; Chassoux *et al.*, 2004; Maillard *et al.*, 2004). Dual pathology associated with hippocampal sclerosis enhances the drug resistance to 97%, while the hippocampal sclerosis alone is already extremely often drug resistant (89% of patients, Semah *et al.*, 1998).

Special remarks

Several studies showed that the experiential phenomena, as complex vivid memory-like recollections, paroxysmal reminiscence, sensations of déjà-vu, and dreamy-state, result from co-activation of medial temporal limbic structures (such as hippocampus and amygdale) and neocortical areas (Halgren *et al.*, 1978; Gloor *et al.*,1982; Bancaud *et al.*, 1994; Bartolomei *et al.*, 2004; Vignal *et al.*, 2007). While the cortical network generating these experiential phenomena was reported by some authors as mainly driven by amygdala and hippocampus (Halgren *et al.*, 1978), more recent studies have proven an important role of the entorhinal and perirhinal cortex by electrical stimulations during invasive depth recordings (Bartolomei *et al.*, 2004). Ictal cephalalgia may have multiple mechanisms (Bernasconi *et al.*, 2001), but sensation of head constriction has been associated with ictal discharges involving the amygdala, or provoked by stimulations in its vicinity (Laplante *et al.*, 1983). This patient had a hippocampal sclerosis, but also a MRI signal abnormality of the amygdala and the anterior

(a)

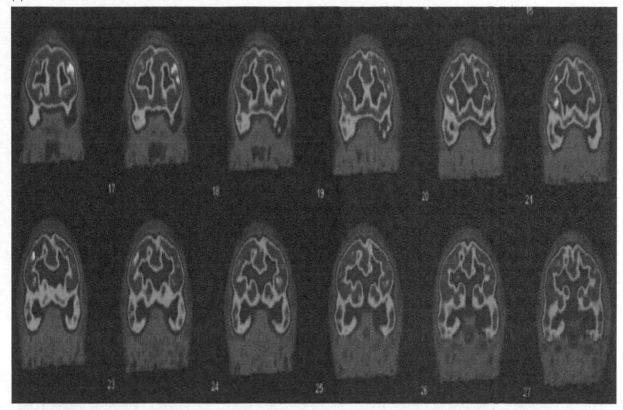

(b)

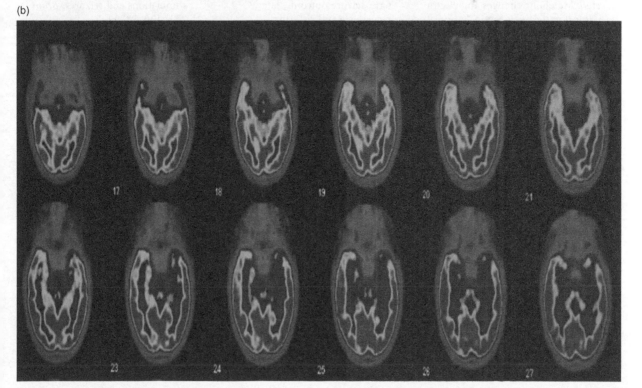

Fig. 5. See color plate section.

rhinal cortex possibly related to an associated focal cortical dysplasia. The electrophysiological data were concordant. Therefore, the experiential phenomena, and later the headache, that the patient reports are very probably generated from the abnormal left amygdala-anterior rhinal region confirming previous studies. However, predominance of non-dominant hemisphere involvement in their production (Vignal *et al.*, 2007) is refuted by the current observation.

Suggested reading

Bancaud J. [Clinical semiology of the seizures of temporal origin]. *Rev Neurol* 1987; **143**: 392–400.

Bancaud J, Brunet-Bourgin F, Chauvel P, Halgren E. Anatomical origin of déjà vu and vivid "memories" in human temporal lobe epilepsy. *Brain* 1994; **117**: 71–90.

Bartolomei F, Barbeau E, Gavaret M, *et al.* Cortical stimulation study of the role of the rhinal cortex in déjà vu and reminiscence of memories. *Neurology* 2004; **63**: 858–64.

Bernasconi A, Andermann F, Bernasconi N, *et al.* Lateralizing value of peri-ictal headache: a study of 100 patients with partial epilepsy. *Neurology* 2001; **56**: 130–2.

Chassoux F, Semah F, Bouilleret V, *et al.* Metabolic changes and electro-clinical patterns in mesio-temporal lobe epilepsy: a correlative study. *Brain* 2004; **127**: 164–74.

Gloor P, Olivier A, Quesney LF *et al.* The role of the limbic system in experiential phenomena of temporal lobe epilepsy. *Ann Neurol* 1982; **12**: 129–44.

Halgren E, Walter RD, Cherlow DG, *et al.* Mental phenomena evoked by electrical stimulation of the human hippocampal formation and amygdala. *Brain* 1978; **101**: 83–117.

Laplante P, Saint-Hilaire JM, Bouvier J. Headache as an epileptic manifestation. *Neurology* 1983; **33**: 1493–5.

Lüders H, Lesser R, Hahn J, *et al.* Basal temporal language area. *Brain* 2001; **114**: 743–54.

McIntosh A, Kalnins R, Mitchell L, *et al.* Temporal lobectomy: long-term seizure outcome, late recurrence and risks for seizure recurrence. *Brain* 2004; **127**: 2018–30.

Pfänder M, Arnold S, Henkel A, *et al.* Clinical features and EEG findings differentiating mesial from neocortical temporal lobe epilepsy. *Epileptic Disord* 2002; **4**: 289–95.

Ray A, Kotagal P. Temporal lobe epilepsy in children: overview of clinical semiology. *Epileptic Disord* 2005; **127**: 164–74.

Semah F, Picot MC, Adam C, *et al.* Is the underlying cause of epilepsy a major prognostic factor for recurrence? *Neurology* 1998; **51**: 1256–62.

Vignal JP, Maillard L, McGonigal A, Chauvel P. The dreamy state: hallucinations of autobiographic memory evoked by temporal lobe stimulations and seizures. *Brain* 2007;**130**: 88–99.

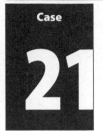

Case

21

The use of depth EEG (SEEG) recordings in a case of frontal lobe epilepsy

Anca Pasnicu, Arnaud Biraben, and Patrick Chauvel

Clinical history

A 14-year-old right-handed boy was referred for pre-surgical evaluation of drug-resistant partial epilepsy. He began to have seizures at the age of three. The seizures were unchanged since the beginning of the epilepsy and they continued despite many antiepileptic drug trials. The patient reported a very brief onset, difficult to describe, as a sensation rapidly ascending from the wrist to the shoulder. Most often he reported this initial sensation in the left upper limb, but sometimes in the right upper limb. The initial sensation was very rapidly followed by sudden left upper limb tonic contraction and lateral abduction, while the right limb seemed to be moving normally. There was also a forward and left version of the head and concomitant deviation of the eyes to the left or to the right. Then there were complex body movements during a dozen seconds. The seizures sometimes stopped or sometimes went on with eyelid rapid myoclonia, then clonic left facio-brachial twitches, and probable laryngeal clonia responsible for rhythmic synchronic moaning. During the seizures the patient had mild late or no loss of consciousness. There was no postictal neurological deficit, but he seemed briefly lost and disoriented, and had a major face flush. Recovery was fast. Only when the seizures were repeated in a cluster did he have gripping difficulties with the left hand and a painful permanent sensation of the entire left upper limb. From the very beginning of the epilepsy, the seizures had been very frequent, up to 20 seizures per day, precipitated by sleep. He had several episodes of partial status epilepticus, but he never had secondary generalized seizures.

General history

Family history was not significant. He had mild asthma and a mild peripheral hypothyroiditis with substitutive treatment. Development had been normal until the epilepsy started. Afterwards, his school attendance was very often disrupted. Because of frequent seizures and learning difficulties, he was constrained to leave the normal school program for an educational establishment for epileptic children.

Examination

General and neurological examinations were normal.

Special studies

During wakefulness, interictal EEG showed few rhythmic slow theta waves over the vertex, mildly lateralized to the right. During sleep there were also central poly-spikes and discharges of spikes, often localized in the right central region (Fig. 1), but at other times it could be maximal over the left central derivations. Three seizures were recorded during video–EEG non-invasive monitoring. Ictal EEG was difficult to analyze because of movement artifacts. At the beginning of the seizures, a rapid discharge was nevertheless apparent over the vertex, on electrode Fz and also on the right pericentral, paramedian regions (Fig. 2).

Neuropsychological assessment

Total and verbal IQ: 68, performance IQ: 69. There was an arrest of the global development, slowness and apathy. There were also memory difficulties, as well as comprehension and attention deficits, but no aphasia. The patient also had calculation deficiency and difficulties in time organization.

Image findings

Cerebral MRI displayed a limited FLAIR hypersignal subcortical in the right mesial frontal area. This

Case Studies in Epilepsy, ed. Hermann Stefan, Elinor Ben-Menachem, Patrick Chauvel and Renzo Guerrini. Published by Cambridge University Press. © Hermann Stefan, Elinor Ben-Menachem, Patrick Chauvel and Renzo Guerrini 2012.

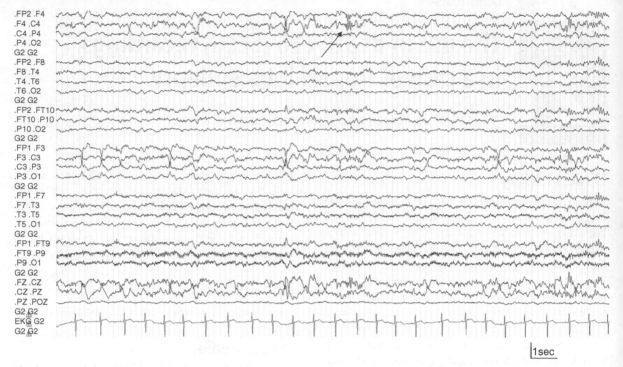

Fig. 1. Interictal sleep EEG: central theta waves and polyspikes (arrow), maximal on the F4-C4 leads (longitudinal montage; FT10, FT9 anterior basal temporal; P10, P9 posterior basal temporal; calibration signal: 1 sec, 100 μV/cm, low filter 0.530 Hz, high filter 120 Hz).

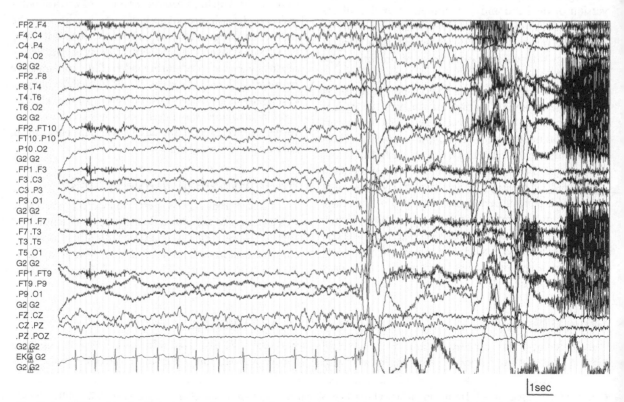

Fig. 2. Ictal EEG: rapid spike discharge over the vertex, on Fz, and also on the right pericentral region at the beginning of the seizure (longitudinal montage; FT10, FT9, P10, P9 see Fig. 1; calibration signal: 1 sec, 100 μV/cm, low filter 0.530 Hz, high filter 120 Hz).

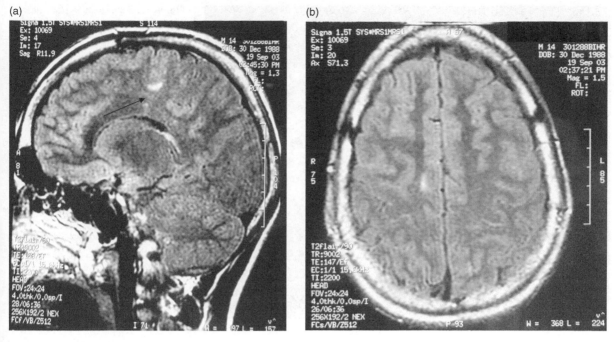

Fig.3. MRI (sagittal and axial FLAIR): subcortical right mesial frontal hypersignal with transmantal sign (arrow).The lesion corresponds to the right SMA region.

subcortical signal abnormality was associated with a transmantal sign, and was localized in the region of the right anterior supplementary motor area (SMA) (Fig. 3). The signal abnormality was not visible in the other MRI sequences. Ictal SPECT showed a large right frontal area of hyperperfusion, from the median polar region to the precentral regions, including the right insula. There was also right lateral frontal and internal temporal hypoperfusion. PET scan is normal.

Stereo-Electroencephalography (SEEG)

Non-invasive electro-clinical data suggested first right pericentral, paramedian epilepsy. The presence of eye movements and the lack of generalized hypertonia suggested that the seizures might originate from the SMA or from the adjacent premotor cortex. The subjective sensation and the early hypertonia of the left upper limb could suggest a postcentral ictal onset. Finally, the left and sometimes right initial subjective sensation and the left and right central paramedian spikes also raised the question of a possible bilateral early involvement. SEEG was performed in order to delineate the ictal onset zone and its relationships with the FLAIR hypersignal right frontal abnormality. We considered that the deep invasive investigation

was also mandatory for functional reasons because of the proximity between the FLAIR hypersignal and the right rolandic region.

Eleven depth electrodes were orthogonally implanted according to the Talairach and Bancaud stereotactic method (Fig. 4).

The conclusion of this SEEG relied upon analysis of the interictal activity, the spontaneous recorded seizures, and the results of electrical stimulations. The medial contacts of electrodes L and Z recorded an interictal activity, which was made up of continuous slow waves and paroxysms without normal background activity (Fig.5). There were spikes, polyspikes, spike-and-wave complexes, and fast discharges, synchronous or not between these two electrodes. The pattern of this activity strongly suggested a focal cortical dysplasia. The spikes and the fast discharges spread to the medial and sometimes intermediary contacts of the electrode R, to the medial contacts of electrode X and to the lateral contacts of the electrodes L and Z, but the interictal background activity remained normal on all these contacts. Therefore, the irritative area and the lesional area overlapped and corresponded to the area explored by the medial contacts of the electrodes L and Z.

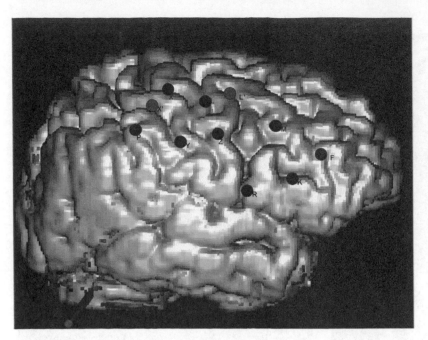

Fig. 4. SEEG implantation plan: the electrodes are orthogonally implanted. Nine electrodes were implanted into the right hemisphere (black dots), they explore from the medial to lateral contacts: **L**: anterior SMA (into the FLAIR signal abnormality) – central fissure – postcentral gyrus; **X**: posterior SMA – precentral gyrus – central fissure – postcentral gyrus; **Y**: posterior cingulate gyrus – postcentral gyrus; **Z**: anterior cingulate gyrus – precentral gyrus; **P**: medial to lateral middle parietal lobe; **M**: preSMA – premotor cortex; **R**: insula – motor operculum; **K**: anterior cingulate gyrus – inferior frontal gyrus; **F**: superior frontal gyrus – middle frontal gyrus. Two electrodes were implanted into the left hemisphere (open dots): **L'**: SMA – premotor cortex; **X'**: medial to lateral superior parietal lobe.

Many seizures were recorded (Fig. 6). They began with an acceleration of the interictal spikes followed by a discharge of rapid spikes, then by a secondary tonic acceleration localized in the medial contacts of electrodes L and Z. This acceleration spread rapidly, but was mildly slower on the lateral contacts of L and Z, on the electrode X (mostly medial), then R (mostly lateral). For most of the seizures, the initial discharge was fastest on the medial contacts of the electrode L, but for some seizures the discharge was fastest on the medial contacts of Z. The seizures recorded during this SEEG were therefore very similar from one to the other but not strictly stereotyped. Moreover, there was a rapid propagation of the tonic discharge on the medial contacts of the electrode X, a region not surgically removable for functional reasons (motor cortex). The ictal onset zone was therefore larger than the irritative and lesional zones, extending more posteriorly and medially, to the primary motor area explored by the medial contacts of X (see below). Finally, the postictal was characterized by a marked but brief slowering limited to the medial contacts of L and Z.

Electrical stimulations by single shocks and by trains of the medial contacts of electrode L provoked electroclinical manifestations resembling the spontaneous seizures. Stimulations of the medial contacts of Z provoked long and high-amplitude after-discharges different from the spontaneous seizures. A functional mapping was performed: no language disturbance was induced by the electrical stimulations of the right-sided electrodes, while the stimulations of the medial contacts of left-sided electrode L induced speech arrest; therefore, the right hemisphere is very likely non-dominant for language; the ictal onset zone corresponds to the right SMA; the stimulations by shocks of the medial contacts of X elicited left inferior limb twitches, demonstrating its location in the leg primary motor area.

Diagnosis

Clinical data together with the non-invasive and invasive electrophysiological recordings, and their correlation with functional and morphological imaging and mapping, enable us to make the diagnosis of right SMA epilepsy related to a probable focal cortical dysplasia, located in a hemisphere non-dominant for language. This conclusion leads to a surgical indication for a cortectomy of the right SMA region, whose boundaries can be determined by the SEEG data. The cortectomy must include the whole MRI right mesial lesion (the area located between the medial contacts of electrodes L and Z) down to the cingulate sulcus on the medial aspect. Dorsally, the cortectomy should extend in front of the area explored by electrode X (posterior dorsal limit) to the region between electrodes L and Z (anterior dorsal limit), up to the superior frontal sulcus (inferior dorsal limit). The area explored by medial contacts of electrode X is part of the ictal onset zone because it

(a)

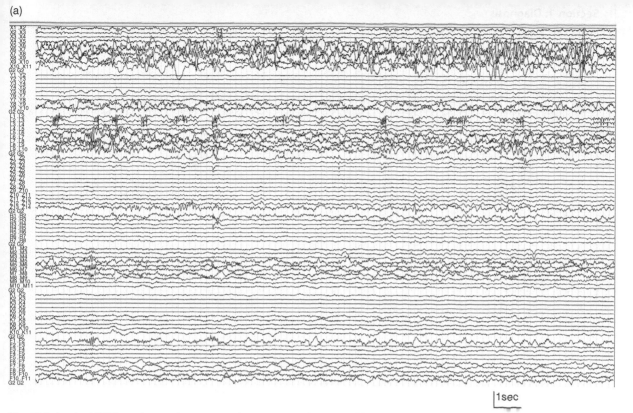

Fig. 5(a). Interictal SEEG: continuous slow waves and paroxysms, and no normal background activity on the medial contacts of electrodes L and Z (bipolar montage; the numbering of the electrodes' contacts starts from the deepest to the most superficial contact; calibration signal: 1 sec, 400 µV/cm, low filter 0.530 Hz, high filter 400 Hz).

(b)

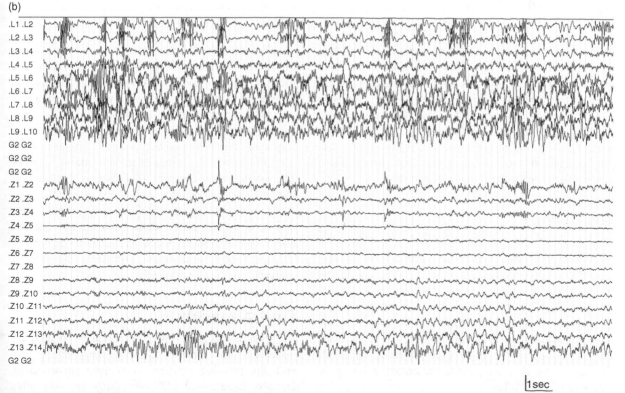

Fig. 5(b). Interictal SEEG: spikes, polyspikes, and discharges of spikes synchronous or not on the medial contacts of L and Z electrodes (bipolar montage; the numbering of the electrodes' contacts see **Fig. 5(a)** calibration signal: 1 sec, 150 µV/cm, low filter 1600 Hz, high filter 400 Hz).

(a)

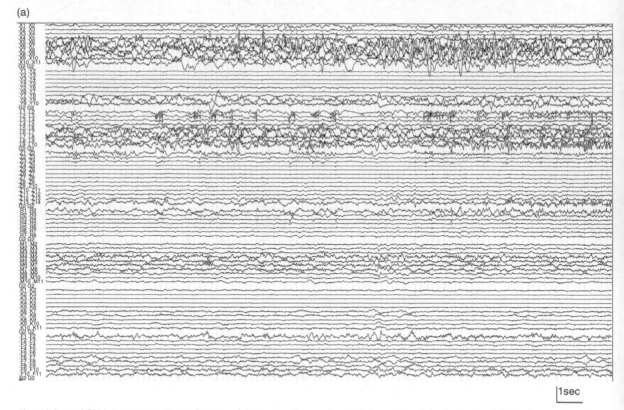

1sec

Fig. 6(a). Ictal SEEG (seizure onset): acceleration of rhythmic spikes on the medial contacts of electrodes L and Z (bipolar montage; the numbering of the electrodes' contacts see Fig. 5a; calibration signal: 1 sec, 400 µV/cm, low filter 0.530 Hz, high filter 400 Hz).

is involved very early by the tonic ictal discharge, but for functional motor reasons it is not removable. This limitation represents a risk factor for seizures recurrence after cortectomy. Nevertheless, this risk isn't major because the interictal activity recorded by the medial contacts of X electrode was consistently normal, in contrast with the one recorded by the medial contacts of L and Z. A transient postoperative left motor hemineglect was anticipated.

Follow-up

The patient was operated on, a few months after SEEG. Pathological examination of the cortex corresponding to the medial contacts of electrodes L and Z confirmed the neuropathological diagnosis of focal cortical dysplasia of Taylor's type. In the immediate postoperative period, the patient had a complete left motor neglect with slight involvement of the face, as expected. The motor neglect decreased at the ninth postoperative day, afterwards the recovery was progressive and complete.

The patient reports that, after the sixth postoperative month, he felt less tired, more active, and that he had more friends at school. Neuropsychological assessment performed 6 months postoperatively showed global improvement of memory, improvement of the visuo-constructive abilities, and of all the fluencies. The other cognitive functions were not modified. The postoperative EEG showed occasional bilateral frontal slow spikes. The postoperative cerebral MRI showed that the cortectomy was performed as it had been planned.

He is now at 7 years of follow-up after cortectomy and he is still on antiepileptic monotherapy. He had only a couple of seizures at 4 years after the surgery in a context of alcohol abuse and sleep deprivation; thereafter he has been seizure free.

General remarks

In this case, SEEG was mandatory principally because of the vicinity of the primary motor area and the possible bilateral early ictal involvement. Invasive intracranial EEG recordings are very often

(b)

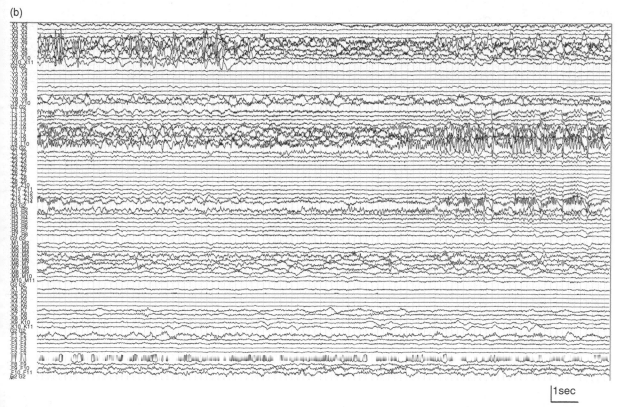

1sec

Fig. 6(b). Ictal SEEG (seizure continued): secondary tonic acceleration which is fastest and the earliest on the medial contacts of electrodes L then Z (red arrows). The tonic discharge diffuses very rapidly on the lateral contacts of L and Z, and also on X, mostly medial (black arrow), and then R, mostly lateral (bipolar montage; the numbering of the electrodes' contacts see Fig. 5(a) calibration signal: 1 sec, 400 µV/cm, low filter 0.530 Hz, high filter 400 Hz).

performed in frontal drug-resistant epilepsies. When epilepsy is cryptogenic or eloquent cortex seems involved early by seizures, intracranial recordings are systematic. Nevertheless, the semiology of the frontal lobe epilepsies is more and more well known, mostly due to the knowledge that was acquired by invasively explored patients (Bancaud, Talairach, 1992; Chauvel *et al.*, 1995; Lüders *et al.*, 1995; Williamson, 1995; Biraben, 2003; Lee *et al.*, 2008). This knowledge progressively enables some of the intracranial EEG recordings to be avoided and a cortectomy to be proposed based on non-invasive data exclusively for selective cases of drug-resistant frontal epilepsies, especially when a lesion is visible and there is no functional risk.

Special remarks

In the patient reported here, the cortectomy was posteriorly bound by the primary motor area for obvious functional reasons. The surgical resection was based on: the non-invasive electroclinical and morphological data, the seizures onset area as identified by the SEEG; and by the SEEG irritative and lesional zones with permanent spikes and faster rhythms and no normal background activity that strongly suggested a focal cortical dysplasia. In these lesions the epileptogenic zone is classically described as corresponding to the irritative and lesional zones (Chassoux *et al.*, 2000). Interictal ripples and fast ripples were also limited to lesional/epileptogenic areas and also were good markers of epileptogenicity (Jacobs *et al.*, 2009, 2010). There were no spikes and fast rhythms, nor background abnormality, in the mesial primary motor area that was, of course, preserved. If there was no eloquent cortex, this area would have been included in the cortectomy because of rapid propagation of the ictal tonic discharge. The fact that this area was preserved might explain why late post-surgical seizures could happen, precipitated by

(c)

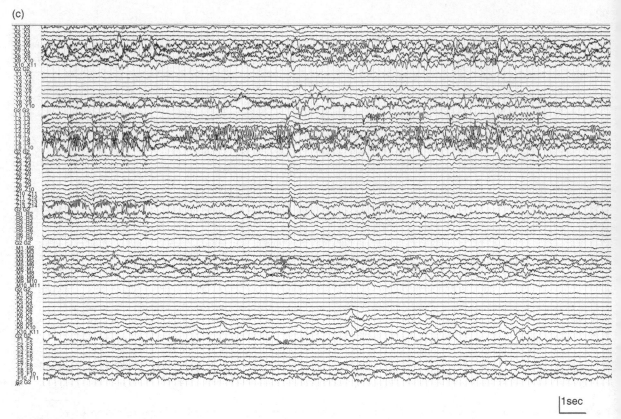

|1sec

Fig. 6(c). Ictal SEEG (seizure end): postictal slowing on the medial contacts of L and Z (bipolar montage; the numbering of the electrodes' contacts see Fig. 5(a) calibration signal: 1 sec, 400 µV/cm, low filter 0.530 Hz, high filter 400 Hz).

alcohol abuse and sleep deprivation. This also explains the need for keeping the patient on an anti-epileptic drug monotherapy.

Future perspectives

When the ictal onset zone is located in eloquent cortex or it is too large to be removed, classical surgery is necessarily limited. In inoperable patients, other validated surgical and stimulation techniques are available, such as multiple subpial transections (Spencer *et al.*,

2002) and vagal nerve stimulation. More recently, subthalamic nucleus stimulation has been reported as an interesting target for deep brain stimulation in primary motor epilepsies (Benabid *et al.*, 2002; Chabardès *et al.*, 2002). Other stimulation targets, especially anterior thalamic nucleus, also seem interesting (Saillet *et al.*, 2009; Fisher *et al.*, 2010). Nevertheless, in non-surgical drug-resistant epilepsies, deep brain stimulation is still a clinical research approach and needs further evaluation.

Suggested reading

Bancaud J, Talairach J. Clinical semiology of frontal lobe seizures. *Adv Neurol* 1992; **57**: 3–58.

Benabid AL, Minotti L, Koudsie A, *et al*. Antiepileptic effect of high-frequency stimulation of the subthalamic nucleus (corpus luysi) in a case of medically intractable

epilepsy caused by focal dysplasia: a 30 month follow-up – technical case report. *Neurosurgery* 2002; **50**: 1385–91.

Biraben A. Classifying the frontal lobe epileptic seizures. *Epileptic Disord* 2003; **5** (Special Issue): SI 27–SI 33.

Chabardès S, Kahane P, Minotti L, *et al*. Deep brain stimulation in

epilepsy with particular reference to the subthalamic nucleus. *Epileptic Disord* 2002; **4**: 83–93.

Chassoux F, Devaux B, Landré E, *et al*. Stereoelectroencephalography in focal cortical dysplasia. A 3D approach to delineating dysplastic cortex. *Brain* 2000; **123**: 1733–551.

Chauvel P, Kliemann F, Vignal JP, *et al.* The clinical signs and symptoms of the frontal lobe seizures. Phenomenology and classification. *Adv Neurol* 1995; **66**: 115–26.

Fisher R, Salanova V, Witt T, *et al.* Electrical stimulation of the anterior nucleus for the treatment of refractory epilepsy. *Epilepsia* 2010; **51**: 899–908.

Jacobs J, LeVan P, Châtillon CE, *et al.* High-frequency oscillations in intracranial EEGs mark epileptogenicity rather than lesion type. *Brain* 2009; **132**: 1022–37.

Jacobs J, Zijlmans M, Zelmann R, *et al.* High-frequency electroencephalographic oscillation correlate with outcome of epilepsy surgery. *Ann Neurol* 2010; **67**: 209–20.

Lee JJ, Lee SK, Lee S-Y, *et al.* Frontal lobe epilepsy: clinical characteristics, surgical outcomes and diagnostic modalities. *Seizure* 2008; **17**: 514–23.

Lüders HO, Dinners DS, Morris HH, *et al.* Cortical electrical stimulation in humans. The negative motor areas. *Adv Neurol* 1995; **67**: 115–29.

Saillet S, Langlois M, Feddersen B, *et al.* Manipulating the epileptic brain using stimulation: a review of the experimental and clinical studies. *Epileptic Disord* 2009; **11**: 1–13.

Spencer SS, Schramm J, Wyler A, *et al.* Multiple subpial transaction for intractable partial epilepsy: an international meta-analysis. *Epilepsia* 2002; **43**: 141–5.

Williamson PD. Frontal lobe epilepsy. Some clinical characteristics. *Adv Neurol* 1995; **66**: 127–52.

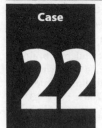

A frontal lobe epilepsy surgery based on totally non-invasive investigations

Martine Gavaret, Jean-Michel Badier, Jean-Claude Peragut, and Patrick Chauvel

Clinical history

A 29-year-old right-handed woman presented with pharmacoresistant partial epilepsy that began at the age of two. The clinical pattern of her seizures did not change over time. The patient described an initial sensation of cardiac acceleration associated with anxiety. Seizures could stop at this moment or continue with intense movements of the body, predominantly axial and proximal, frightened expression, vocalization, mydriasis, and facial flushing. There was apparently no loss of consciousness. Seizures had a nocturnal predominance, occurred in clusters, and were characterized by a short duration, lasting 10 to 40 seconds. Secondary generalization was rare. There was no family history of epilepsy.

Examination

Physical and neurological examinations were normal. Neuropsychological examination highlighted a dysexecutive syndrome with deficit of verbal inhibition, difficulties in strategy planning and problem resolution, with a tendency to perseveration.

Special studies:

Video-EEG recording: Several seizures were recorded. Clinically, the patient described a sensation of cardiac acceleration then presented intense stereotypical movements of flexion of both legs on the trunk and anteflexion of the trunk, with an elementary vocalization, a bilateral facial contraction and at certain moments, a frightened expression. Seizures were very brief, lasting 18-20 seconds and were characterized by immediate recovery. Ictal EEG was characterized by initial high amplitude ictal spikes, being of maximal amplitude on channels FP2, F8, F4, Fz, FP1 (monopolar montage, common average reference). (fig. 1)

High resolution EEG: A: Surface interictal spikes were recorded with 64 channels and a 1000 Hz sampling rate. Their amplitude was maximal on channels FP2, F8, F10, F4 (monopolar montage, common average reference). **B:** Amplitude cartography (using Focus soft-ware) during the single interictal spike marked by the vertical line in panel A. **C:** The same single interictal spike, 64 channels superimposed. The temporal window of analysis lies between the two vertical lines. **D:** Electrode positions, patient's head contour and 3D-MRI had the same spatial reference and were superimposed. The realistic head model, based on a boundary element method, is elaborated using the patient's 3D MRI (detailed methodology in Gavaret et al, 2006). **E:** Interictal source localizations using MUSIC (ASA soft-ware) were localized in the right anterior lateral frontal lobe, around the intermediate frontal sulcus (axial and coronal slices) (fig 2).

A: Magnetoencephalography (MEG): Interictal spikes were recorded with a 151-channel MEG system (CTF Systems Inc., Port Coquitlam, Canada). MEG amplitude cartography during the interictal spikes marked by vertical lines. **B:** MEG source localizations were performed using a spatio-temporal fit approach (Schwartz et al, 2003) and indicated the region of the right intermediate frontal sulcus. **C: Pre-operative cerebral MRI:** Gyral thickening of the right intermediate frontal sulcus, with abnormal MRI signal, was suggestive of focal cortical dysplasia according to the criteria of Kuzniecky & Barkovich, 2001 (fig. 3).

PET was not performed. Based on the electroclinical features, high resolution EEG, MEG and MRI data, epilepsy surgery consisting of a resection of the right intermediate frontal sulcus was planned. Anatomo-pathological examination demonstrated

---

Case Studies in Epilepsy, ed. Hermann Stefan, Elinor Ben-Menachem, Patrick Chauvel and Renzo Guerrini. Published by Cambridge University Press. © Hermann Stefan, Elinor Ben-Menachem, Patrick Chauvel and Renzo Guerrini 2012.

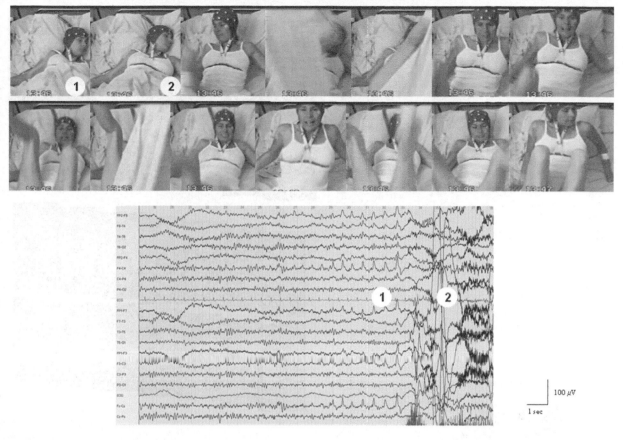

Fig. 1. Video-EEG recording: ictal EEG was characterized by initial high amplitude ictal spikes, being of maximal amplitude on channels FP2, F8, F4, F2, FP1 (monopolar mortage, common average spikes). See color plate section.

Taylor focal cortical dysplasia type IIB (architectural abnormalities with dysmorphic neurons and balloon cells) (Palmini et al, 2004). Post-operative cerebral MRI (axial slices) (fig. 4).

Follow-up

At the time of writing, the patient has been seizure free for 6 years. She has had no antiepileptic treatment for the past 4 years. Neuropsychological examination is improved with reduced impulsiveness and improved planning strategies.

General remarks

This case is a rare case of pharmacoresistant and severe frontal lobe epilepsy operated without intracerebral investigations. This decision was taken because all non-invasive electrophysiological data were coherent, indicating the same region of the right intermediate frontal sulcus where a focal cortical dysplasia was secondarily highlighted by the MRI. We noticed that ictal scalp EEG demonstrated repetitive spikes of high amplitude, which were comparable to interictal spikes. It is likely in these cases of ictal spiking, related to focal cortical dysplasia, indicating a congruence of epileptogenic and primary irritative zones, that the contribution of HR-EEG and MEG interictal source localizations is maximal among all presurgical investigations (Chauvel *et al.*, 1987; Palmini *et al.*, 1995; Chassoux *et al.*, 2000).

Without this lesion and interictal source localizations, we would not have deduced, according to the semiology, that the epilepsy was organized in this region of the intermediate frontal sulcus. Indeed, the initial sensation of cardiac acceleration and intense

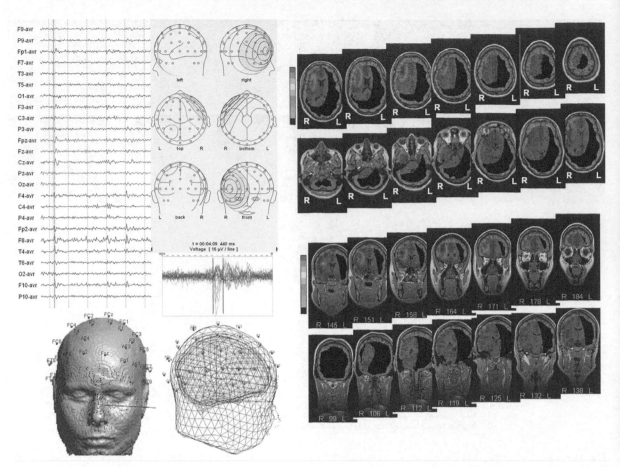

Fig. 2. High resolution EEG: Surface interictal spikes were recorded with 64 channels and a Hz sampling rate as well as amplitude cartography (using focus software). See color plate section.

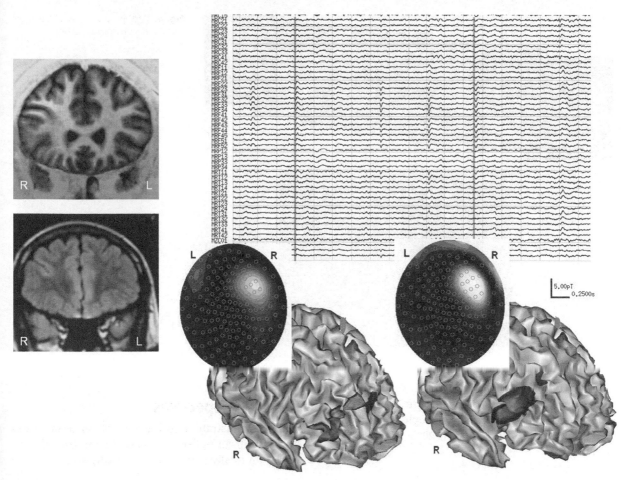

Fig. 3. A: Magnetoencephalography (MEG); B: MWG source localization; C: preoperative MRI. See color plate section.

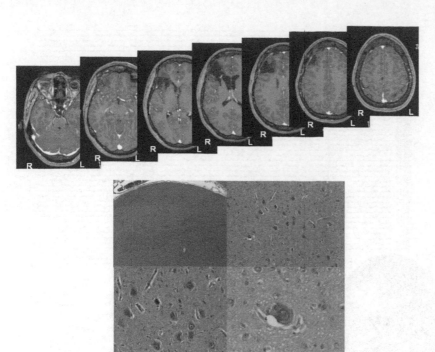

Fig. 4. Postoperative cerebral MRI (axial slices). See color plate section.

stereotypical movements were more evocative of a mesio-ventral or temporo-frontal implication (Bancaud and Talairach, 1992; Chauvel, 2003; Vaugier *et al.*, 2009).

Future perspectives

This case illustrates that it is possible in certain cases to perform an epilepsy surgery, in the frontal lobe, based on totally non-invasive investigations.

Suggested reading

Bancaud J, Talairach J. Clinical semiology of frontal lobe seizures. *Adv Neurol* 1992; **57**: 3–58.

Chassoux F, Devaux B, Landre E, *et al.* Stereoelectroencephalography in focal cortical dysplasia: a 3D approach to delineating the dysplastic cortex. *Brain* 2000; **123**: 1733–51.

Chauvel P. Can we classify frontal lobe seizures? In A Beaumanoir, F Andermann, P Chauvel, L Mira, B Zifkin, eds. *Frontal Seizures and Epilepsies in Children.* John Libbey Eurotext, 2003, 59–64.

Chauvel P, Buser P, Badier JM, *et al.* La «zone épileptogène» chez l'homme: représentation des événements intercritiques par cartes spatio-temporelles. *Rev Neurol* 1987; **143**: 443–50.

Gavaret M, Badier JM, Marquis P, *et al.* Electric source imaging in frontal lobe epilepsy. *Journal of Clinical Neurophysiology* 2006; **23**: 358–70.

Kuzniecky RI, Barkovich AJ. Malformations of cortical development and epilepsy. *Brain Dev* 2001; **23**: 2–11.

Palmini A, Gambardella A, Andermann F, *et al.* Intrinsic epileptogenicity of human dysplastic cortex as suggested by corticography and surgical results. *Ann Neurol* 1995; **37**: 476–87.

Palmini A, Najm I, Avanzini G, *et al.* Terminology and classification of the cortical dysplasias. *Neurology* 2004; **62**: S2–8.

Schwartz DP, Badier JM, Vignal JP, *et al.* Non-supervised spatio-temporal analysis of interictal magnetic spikes: comparison with intracerebral recordings. *Clin Neurophysiol* 2003; **114**: 438–49.

Vaugier L, Aubert S, McGonigal A, *et al.* Neural networks underlying hyperkinetic seizures of "temporal lobe" origin. *Epilepsy Res* 2009; **86**: 200–8.

Case
23
A young man with reading-induced seizure

Anne Thiriaux, Nathalie Ehrle, Jean-Pierre Vignal,
Louis Maillard, and Audrey Henry

Clinical history

A 36-year-old right-handed French patient was admitted for a generalized tonic–clonic seizure (GTCS). While reading aloud an English text, his jaw started jerking and he could no longer understand what he was reading, his vision became clouded, then he fell to the ground with a GTCS. Since the age of 15, he had noticed episodes of jerks involving the jaw when reading and also speaking, especially when he was tired. He probably presented a first GTCS 10 years ago. At this time, he was reading a French text for more than 10 minutes, when he experienced orofacial myoclonia. He was unable to understand the sentence's meaning and then had a loss of consciousness. He was alone, and woke up later with cephalalgia.

Precipitating factors

The jaw jerks were triggered by stress, weariness, alcohol, or cannabis intake.

General history

There was no personal or family history, apart from bronchial asthma. He had particularly good acquisition of reading skills; he started to read at 4 years old.

Examination

The physical and neurological examinations were normal.

Electroencephalography

A first interictal EEG with hyperventilation and photic stimulation according to the international 10–20 system of electrode placement was normal.

A prolonged video–EEG monitoring was performed according to the international 10–20 system of electrode with perioral EMG. Speaking and reading during continuous video–EEG monitoring provoked myoclonia. Ictal EEG showed brief diffuse sharp theta wave discharges associated with reading or speaking induced jaw jerking. The sharp theta wave discharges were predominantly seen on the left side.

Reading aloud provoked more myoclonia than reading silently. Texts written in a foreign language or with more difficulties (irregular words or pseudo-words, for example) were more precipitating factors. The patient had myoclonia when he was only speaking, but had no myoclonia when he was only writing.

Image findings

The cerebral MRI was normal.

Neuropsychological assessment

The patient had a normal efficiency (GIQ: 111, shortened form of the French version of the Wechsler Adult Intelligence Scale-Revised, WAIS-R), without any significant dissociation between verbal (VIQ: 109) and performance IQ (PIQ: 107). His episodic memory performances were in the normal range, for both verbal (California Verbal Learning Test) and visual stimuli (Rey–Osterrieth Complex Figure). The examination of language did not demonstrate any naming, reading, writing, understanding, or fluency deficit (French version of the Boston Naming Test, Chapman–Cook Speed of Reading Test). His spontaneous expression was considered both formally and semantically rich.

Diagnosis

The history, the video–EEG data with the precipitating factors evoking paroxysmal activities (Fig. 1),

---

Case Studies in Epilepsy, ed. Hermann Stefan, Elinor Ben-Menachem, Patrick Chauvel and Renzo Guerrini. Published by Cambridge University Press. © Hermann Stefan, Elinor Ben-Menachem, Patrick Chauvel and Renzo Guerrini 2012.

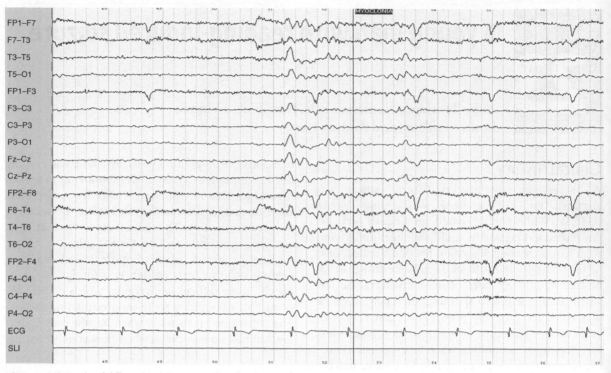

Fig. 1. Ictal EEG: brief diffuse sharp theta wave discharges with left side predominance. They are associated with jaw jerks.

associated with a normal MRI allowed us to make the diagnosis of reading epilepsy.

Treatment and evolution

The patient tried treatment with sodium valproate. He was only partially controlled (less frequent myoclonia and no more GTCS). He decided to stop treatment because of adverse events. He avoided precipitating factors and took 1 mg of clonazepam if necessary (if more myoclonia when he was tired or when he had to make oral presentation or to read longer...). He never had GTCS any more (6 years follow-up).

Commentary

Reflex epilepsy is a condition in which seizures can be precipitated by an external or an internal stimulus.

Reading epilepsy was first described by Bickford *et al.* (1956) who reported mouth jerking possibly followed by generalization provoked by reading in eight patients. The characteristics of these epilepsies are heterogeneous. Koutroumanidis *et al.* (1998) identified two types of reading epilepsy: myoclonic reading epilepsy and partial reading epilepsy. In the

myoclonic reading epilepsy, seizures begin with jaw jerks without alexia, accompanied by bilateral EEG paroxysms more or less lateralized to the left. The seizures are often provoked by other stimuli, mainly speech. A history of myoclonic epilepsy is frequent (Radhakrishnan *et al.*, 1995). More rarely, partial reading seizures begin with alexia and are associated with left or bilateral independent temporal ictal discharges (Maillard *et al.*, 2010). Our patient presents the first type. In this case, the ictal manifestations are often jaw jerks that can evolve into GTCS if reading is continued. In our case, reading and talking triggered the myoclonia. Interictal EEG may be normal as reported in our patient and in 80% of previously published cases (Wolf, 1992). Reading evokes brief spike/sharp-wave discharges or theta wave discharges on EEG associated with the induced jaw jerkings. Sometimes, jerks occur without any EEG modification. Paroxysmal EEG abnormalities are bilateral and symmetrical in one-third of cases and bilateral with a left side predominance in another one-third of patients (Wolf, 1992). Myoclonic reading epilepsy usually starts in adolescence or young adulthood. The age at onset is 17.7 years on average (Wolf, 1992). Neurological examination intelligence quotient and cerebral MRI are usually normal. Lesional cases are rare and involve left temporal or frontal lobe. Four cases of myoclonic reading epilepsy were reported in left hemisphere strokes (Bickford et al., 1956; Lee et al., 1980; Radhakrishnan et al., 1995; Koutroumanidis et al., 1998), and one case of arterio-venous malformation in the left frontal lobe (Ritaccio et al., 1992) A family history of epilepsy is found in 41% of cases with 11 cases among 20 of reading epilepsy in relectures (Wolf, 1992). There is a male predominance with 13 men vs. 7 women in Radhakrishnan et al. (1995) and 12 men vs. 5 women in Koutroumanidis et al. (1998). Myoclonic reading epilepsy is usually treated by clonazepam, valproate, topiramate, or levetiracetam and the outcome is usually favorable.

What did we learn from these cases?

Reading epilepsy is rare and may appear as anecdotal. However, it should be considered in the light of a very interesting study reporting paroxysmal discharges evoked by cognitive tasks in 38 out of 480 Japanese patients with epilepsy (8%). Among these 38 patients, 36 had generalized epilepsy, with a majority of myoclonic generalized epilepsy (Matsuoka et al., 2000). The triggering tasks were writing, visuo-spatial construction tasks, written and mental arithmetic, and reading. All new suspected cases of generalized seizure should be asked for a cognitive triggering factor.

Suggested reading

Bickford RG, Whelan JL, Klass DW, Corbin KB. Reading epilepsy: clinical and electroencephalographic studies of a new syndrome. *Trans Am Neurol Assoc* 1956; **81**: 100–2.

Koepp MJ, Hansen ML, Pressler RM et al. Comparison of EEG, MRI and PET in reading epilepsy: a case report. *Epilepsy Res* 1998; **29**: 251–7.

Koutroumanidis M, Koepp MJ, Richardson MP, Camfield C. The variants of reading epilepsy: a clinical and video-EEG study of 17 patients with reading-induced seizures. *Brain* 1998; **121**: 1409–27.

Lee SJ, Sutherling WW, Persing JA, Butler AB. Language-induced seizure. A case of cortical origin. *Arch Neurol* 1980; **37**: 433–6.

Maillard L, Vignal JP, Raffo E, Vespignani H. Bitemporal form of partial reading epilepsy: further

evidence for an idiopathic localization-related syndrome. *Epilepsia* 2010; **51**:165–9.

Matsuoka H, Takahashi T, Sasaki M, et al. Neuropsychological EEG activation in patients with epilepsy. *Brain* 2000; **123**: 318–30.

Radhakrishnan K, Silbert PL, Klass DW. Reading epilepsy: an appraisal of 20 patients diagnosed at the Mayo Clinic Rochester, Minnesota, between 1949 and 1989, and delineation of the epileptic syndrome. *Brain* 1995; **118**: 75–89.

Ritaccio AL, Hicking EJ, Ramani V. The role of dominant premotor cortex and grapheme to phoneme transformation in reading epilepsy: a neuroanatomic, neurophysiologic and neuropsychological study. *Arch Neurol* 1992; **49**: 933–9.

Singh B, Anderson L, Al Gashlan M, Al-Shahwan SA, Riela AR.

Reading-induced absence seizures. *Neurology* 1995; **45**: 1623–24.

Wolf P. L'épilepsie à la lecture. In J Roger, Ch Dravet, FE Dreifuss, A Perret, P Wolf, eds. *Les syndromes épileptiques de l'enfant et de l'adolescent*. London: John Libbey & Co Ltd, 1992, 2nd edn., 281–90.

Wolf P, Inoue Y. Epilepsies réflexes complexes: épilepsie de la lecture et crises induites par des praxies ("praxis induction"). In J Roger, M Bureau, P Dravet, et al., eds. *Les Syndromes Epileptiques de l'Enfant et de l'Adolescent*. London: John Libbey & Co Ltd, 2005, 4th edn., 347–58.

Wolf P, Mayer T, Reker M. Reading epilepsy: report of five new cases and further consideration on the pathophysiology. *Seizure* 1996; **7**: 271–9.

Yalçin AD, Forta H. Primary reading epilepsy. *Seizure* 1998; **7**: 325–7.

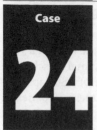

Case

24

The lady from "no-man's-land"

Friedhelm C. Schmitt and Stefan Rampp

Clinical history

The 31-year-old, right-handed female patient presented with repeated episodes of staring and diminished responsiveness over several minutes up to hours. Currently, these episodes occur one to three times daily. Similar spells of much shorter duration (several minutes) had been observed, when the patient was a school child. At that time grand mal seizures were reported and antiepileptic drug (AED) medication initiated. Since then, at least nine AEDs have been used without a considerable reduction of seizure frequency. The actual medication was reliably taken (topiramate 300 mg/day and lamotrigine 300 mg/day).

General history

Birth, further child development, past medical and family history were unremarkable.

Examination

During an observed episode she had her eyes open, but could not comply to easy, straightforward challenges. Automated actions, such as counting and walking, were performed easily. After the episode, the patient could neither recall her own activities nor the challenges she had been exposed to. She was her "usual self" and would converse without any difficulties. Besides impaired consciousness, she did not have clinical signs in the neurological examination.

Neurological scores on admission

Glasgow Coma Scale: Patient opens eyes spontaneously (4 points), is verbally confused and disoriented (4 points), and localizes painful stimuli in motor test (5 points).

Special studies

Repeated MRIs were reported to be normal, routine EEG showed discrete bitemporal slowing and rarely posteriorly accentuated generalized trains of sharp waves over 2–5 seconds.

Follow-up

A presurgical work-up with long-term video–EEG monitoring, 3-tesla MRI and interictal/ictal MEG was advised.

The long-term video–EEG monitoring revealed a bitemporo-occipital seizure pattern over hours (roughly 6–10 hours) per day (Fig. 1) sometimes interrupted by left temporo-lateral (Fig. 2) or bitemporal (left more often than right) sharp waves (Fig. 3). The seizure pattern coincided with the above described epidodes up to four times a day.

A 3-tesla MRI including a voxel-based morphometry was normal and a MEG study was performed for further localization (see below).

Image findings (Figs. 4–5)

Diagnosis

Pharmacoresistant, non-lesional epilepsy with repetitive non-convulsive status epilepticus, allegedly from the left temporo-lateral region.

General remarks

Already in the nineteenth century physicians had described non-convulsive status epilepticus (NCSE). A similar episode as in the presented case with preserved automated locomotion was reported as early as Charcot 1888 by (Shorvon, 1994) (Figure 6).

Case Studies in Epilepsy, ed. Hermann Stefan, Elinor Ben-Menachem, Patrick Chauvel and Renzo Guerrini. Published by Cambridge University Press. © Hermann Stefan, Elinor Ben-Menachem, Patrick Chauvel and Renzo Guerrini 2012.

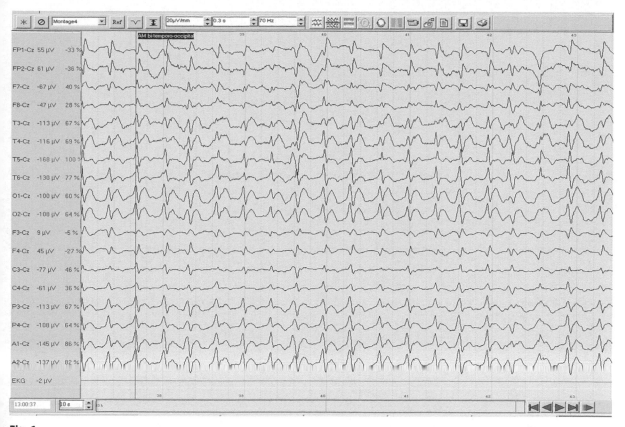

Fig. 1.

In some cases the duration of NCSE is reported to sustain for weeks to years. Differential diagnosis of NCSE is numerous and includes prolonged post-ictal confusion, metabolic encephalopathy, substance de- or intoxication, transient global amnesia, and status migranicus. Also, clinical presentation of NCSE varies, depends on the underlying pathology, and is not pathognomic *per se*. Therefore, ictal EEG recordings should be performed to support the diagnosis of NCSE. Clinical presentation, ictal EEG, and underlying etiology determine the classification and subsequent treatment options of different types of NCSE (Meierkord and Holtkamp, 2007). Generally, first- and second-line treatment should be administered as early as possible, but there is considerable agreement to refrain from aggressive treatment such as anesthetic anticonvulsants, because the risk of this treatments outweighs its putative benefit (EFNS Guidelines, 2010).

Special remarks

In spite of several AED regimens, the presented patient has a high frequency of repeated NCSE. She was considerably impaired in her everyday activity and pursuit of life. All reasonable and available diagnostic tools for a presurgical work-up should be considered. Patients with non-lesional MRI have a 2.5 to 2.9-fold risk not to obtain seizure freedom in comparison to patients with lesional MRI findings (Téllez-Zenteno *et al.*, 2010). However, for resective surgery a reliable localization of the putative epileptogenic zone is crucial. MEG can add further important information for a better localization, as it has been proven both for ictal and interictal MEG recordings (Eliashiv, *et al.*, 2002; Stefan *et al.*, 1992, Sutherling *et al.*, 1987).

On the basis of the findings of the MEG, this patient can be offered further presurgical diagnostic evaluation such as invasive EEG monitoring.

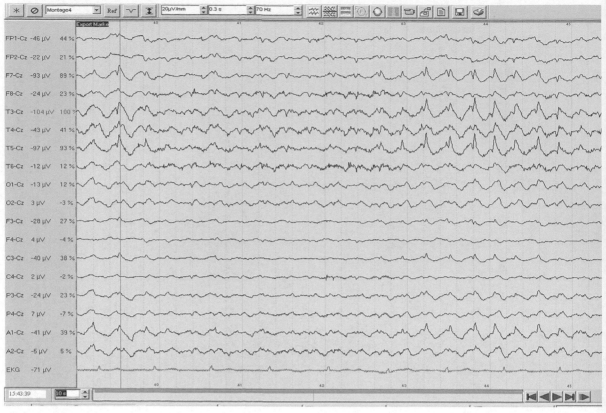

Fig. 2.

Suggested reading

Eliashiv DS, Elsas SM, Squires K, Fried I, Engel J, Jr. Ictal magnetic source imaging as a localizing tool in partial epilepsy. *Neurology* 2002; **59**: 1600–10.

Meierkord H, Holtkamp M. Non-convulsive status epilepticus in adults: clinical forms and treatment. *Lancet Neurol* 2007; **6**: 329–39.

Meierkord H, Boon P, Engelsen B, *et al.* EFNS guideline on the management of status epilepticus in adults. *Eur J Neurol* 2010; **17**: 348–55.

Shorvon S. *Status Epilepticus: Its Clinical Features and Treatment in Children and Adults.* Cambridge: Cambridge University Press, 1994.

Stefan H, Schneider S, Feistel H. Ictal and interictal activity in partial epilepsy recorded with multichannel magnetoelectroencephalography: correlation of electroencephalography/ electrocorticography, magnetic resonance imaging, single photon emission computed tomography, and positron emission tomography findings. *Epilepsia* 1992; **33**: 874–87.

Stefan H, Rampp S, Knowlton RC. Magnetoencephalography adds to surgical evaluation process. *Epilepsy Behav* 2011; **20**: 172–7.

Sutherling WW, Crandall PH, Engel J Jr, *et al.* The magnetic field of complex partial seizures agrees with intracranial localizations. *Ann Neurol* 1987; **21**: 548–58.

Téllez-Zenteno JF, Hernández Ronquillo L, Moien-Afshari F, Wiebe S. Surgical outcomes in lesional and non-lesional epilepsy: a systematic review and meta-analysis. *Epilepsy Res* 2010; **89**: 310–18.

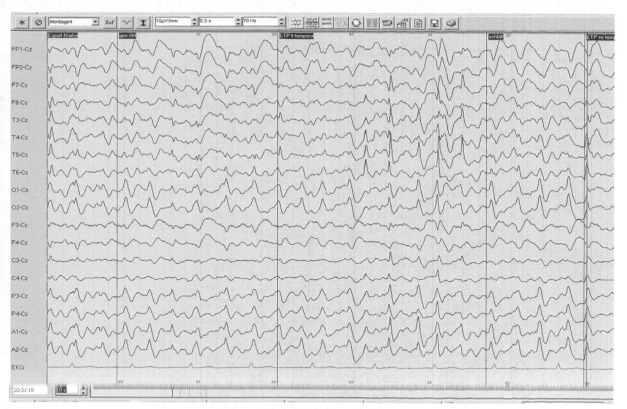

Fig. 3.

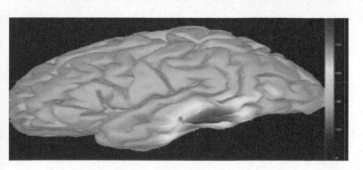

Fig. 4. MSI (MRI coregistered with MEG-dipole localisation): dipole analysis of the ictal MEG showed focal spike formation (red) in the left temporal region (infrasylvic, at the posterior portions of the superior and medial temporal gyri and posteriorly to the angular gyrus). See color plate section.

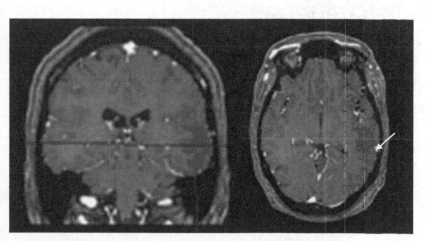

Fig. 5. The averaged dipole analysis (LORETA-analysis with interictal MEG) revealed a similar localization. See color plate section.

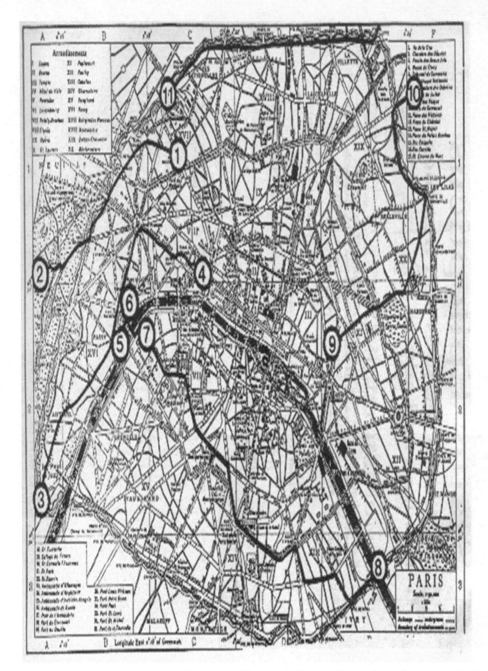

Fig. 6. Charcot described the route of a 37-year-old man with "fugue epileptique", wandering around in Paris for days without recollection of so doing (From Shorvon, 1994.)

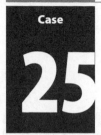

Case

25

The man who came (too) late

Friedhelm C. Schmitt

Clinical history

This 56-year-old, right-handed male patient has had complex focal seizures since the age of three. Rarely, he reported an aura with an unspecific feeling that "there was something coming up." His parents reported that seizures started usually with fidgeting and unresponsiveness; sometimes he would senselessly continue the action he was doing before the seizure. Occasionally, seizures would develop to "heavy shaking of the body." Then, he had a prolonged postictal confusion, tongue bite, and myalgia. There has been no prolonged period of seizure freedom in his life, even though he has received adequate medical treatment; he has taken seven appropriately dosed and well-tolerated antiepileptic drugs without a significant effect on his habitual seizure frequency of two to six complex focal seizures per month. Concise evaluation of the drug history showed that a partial anti-ictal effect was attributable to carbamazepine (reduction led reversibly to an increase of seizure frequency, which could not be explained by pharmacokinetic drug interaction). Five AEDs (PHT, PRM, GBP, PRG and TGB) have been taken in the past without reaching adequate dosage. Current medication was zonisamide 400 mg/day, carbamazepine 900 mg/day, and levetiracetam 2000 mg/day.

The patient worked as a saddler and upholsterer until the age of 37, since then he has been unemployed. He has always lived with his parents in a rural area, is unmarried, and has no children. Because of continuous seizures, he has no driving licence.

General history

Birth was unremarkable. The first seizures occurred during an unspecific febrile disease at the age of three. At 11 years old, he had an uncomplicated appendectomy. Besides an arterial hypertension, he has had no other remarkable disease, including cerebral vascular events.

Examination

He had bilateral palmomental reflexes. Otherwise, no clinical signs – including gait and muscle tone – were detected. During the explorative interview, no memory deficits became evident; however, the patient seemed slightly deferred in his communicative reaction and mimic expression. There were no complaints or symptoms of depression.

Neurological scores on admission

Special studies

Routine EEG showed a mild generalized intermitting generalized slowing, left fronto-temporal and right temporo-lateral slowing, and left fronto-temporal spikes

Follow-up

A presurgical work-up with long-term video–EEG monitoring, MRI with hippocampal angulation, interictal SPECT, and neuropsychological testing was advised.

During the long-term video–EEG monitoring, six habitual complex focal (semiological classification: automotor) seizures with a corresponding left anterotemporal (five times) or left hemispheric (once) seizure pattern were detected. Interictal spikes were exclusively left fronto-temporal with a rather high frequency (approx. 35 spikes/10 minutes) and a clear preponderance during sleep (3 to 1) (see Fig. 1 and Fig. 2).

MRI and interictal SPECT – see below.

In a detailed neuropsychological testing the patient showed pronounced deficits in executive functions, cognitive flexibility, and figural memory. Verbal memory functions were normal.

Case Studies in Epilepsy, ed. Hermann Stefan, Elinor Ben-Menachem, Patrick Chauvel and Renzo Guerrini. Published by Cambridge University Press. © Hermann Stefan, Elinor Ben-Menachem, Patrick Chauvel and Renzo Guerrini 2012.

Image findings (Figs. 1, 2)

Coronal view from FLAIR-MRI: abnormal are the hyperintense, hypotrophy, left hippocampal structure (see arrow) and the multiple, diffuse, infra- and supratentorial subcortical hyperintensities.

Coronal view of interictal SPECT (740 MbQ-Tc-99 m) with hypoperfusion of left temporal lobe (see arrows).

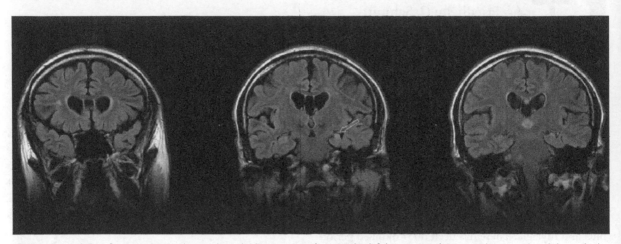

Fig. 1. Coronal view from FLAIR-MRI: abnormal are the hyperintense, hypotrophy, left hippocampal structure (see arrow) and the multiple, diffuse, infra- and supratentorial subcortical hyperintensities.

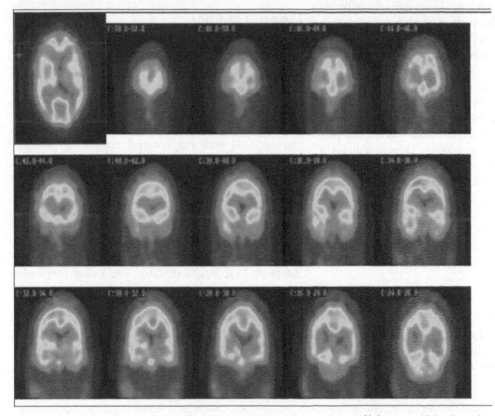

Fig. 2. Coronal view of interictal SPECT (740 MbQ-Tc-99m) with hypoperfusion of left temperal lobe. See color plate section.

Diagnosis

1. Pharmacoresistant epilepsy with unspecific auras, complex focal seizures, and grand mal from the left temporal lobe.
2. Left hippocampal sclerosis.
3. Vascular encephalopathy.

General remarks

The patient and his parents describe clearly a long-term medical history with unspecific auras, complex seizures and occasional grand mal seizures. The ictal seizure pattern, postictal SPECT, and the MRI confirm the diagnosis of left temporal lobe epilepsy due to hippocampal sclerosis. The social impact of this patient's epilepsy has been profound: he has been unemployed for almost two decades. Living in the rural area with restricted public transportation, his means of independent travelling are constrained and he lives as a bachelor in the house of his aging parents.

Resective epilepsy surgery is the treatment of choice in pharmacoresistant temporal lobe epilepsy with concordant findings in the presurgical diagnostic work-up. Postsurgical outcome proved to be highly superior to medical treatment (Schmidt and Stavem, 2009; Wiebe et al., 2001). This procedure should be considered as soon as medical treatment has not achieved seizure freedom and formal pharmacoresistance is attained (Kwan et al., 2011). As in the presented patient, video-monitoring – the key diagnostic tool in the presurgical work-up (Rosenow and Lueders, 2001) – is often conducted belatedly. For a decade, the mean duration of epilepsy prior to temporal lobe epilepsy has remained unchanged at 20 years (Choi et al., 2009). Even though elderly patients with temporal lobe epilepsy seem to have a similar postoperative outcome concerning seizure outcome, the risk of complications is elevated (Srikijvilaikul et al., 2011; Stefan, 2011) and lower neuropsychological performance anticipated (Stefan, 2011).

Special remarks

The latter concern should receive additional consideration in the presented patient, since he might have additional neuropsychological impairment by the vascular encephalopathy, which is suggested by examination, past medical history, and MRI. The neuropsychological deficit comprises figural memory and predominant frontal lobe functions. Notably, there was no deficit in verbal memory in the presented case, even though this would be expected in a right handed patient with left temporal lobe epilepsy pertinent since early childhood. Concerning the intact verbal memory, it can be reasonably speculated that there was a total or partial shift of language function due to the life-long functional impairment in the epileptogenic left temporal lobe, an effect well known in temporal lobe epilepsy patients (Moeddel et al., 2009).

Future perspectives

For certain epilepsy patients who are not straightforward candidates for resective surgery, other surgical techniques have been discussed. Stereotactically guided radiofrequency lesioning is a minimal invasive technique, which allows preservation of overlying cortex and – in case of negative results – possible reapplication or later realization of resective surgery. In a small series of patients with temporal lobe epilepsy, 1-year-postoperative seizure outcome was comparable to resective surgery (Kalina et al., 2007).

Suggested reading

Choi H, Carlino R, Heiman G, Hauser WA, Gilliam F G. Changes in time to temporal lobe epilepsy surgery. Epilepsy Res 2009; 86: 224–7.

Kalina M, Lisck R, Vojtech Z, et al. Stereotactic amygdalohippokampectomy for temporal lobe epilepsy: promising results in 16 patients, Epileptic Disorder 2007; 9: S68–S74.

Kwan P, Schachter SC, Brodie MJ. Drug-resistant epilepsy, N Engl J Med 2011; 8: 919–26.

Moeddel G, Lineweaver T, Schuele SU, Reinholz J, Loddenkemper T. Atypical language lateralization in epilepsy patients. Epilepsia 2009; 50: 1505–16.

Rosenow F, Lueders H. Presurgical evaluation of epilepsy. Brain 2001; 124: 1683–700.

Schmidt D, Stavem K. Long-term seizure outcome of surgery versus no surgery for drug-resistant partial epilepsy: a review of controlled studies. Epilepsia 2009; 50: 1301–9.

Srikijvilaikul T, Lerdlum S, Tepmongkol S, Shuangshoti S,

Locharernkul C. Outcome of temporal lobectomy for hippocampal sclerosis in older patients. *Seizure* 2011; **20**, 276–9.

Stefan H. Epilepsy in the elderly: facts and challenges. *Acta Neurol Scand* 2011; **124**: 223–37.

Wiebe S, Blume WT, Girvin JP, *et al*. A randomized controlled trial of surgery for temporal lobe epilepsy. *N Engl J Med* 2001; **345**: 311–18.

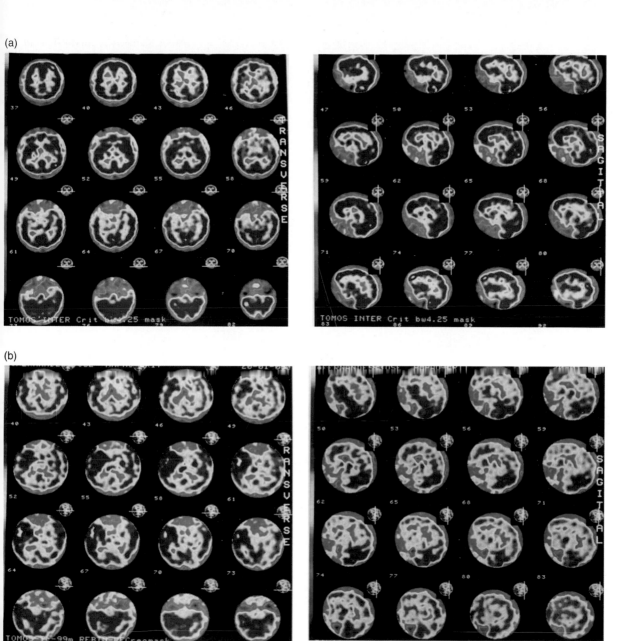

Fig. 19.4. Interictal SPECT (**a**): hypoperfusion of the right temporal pole and of the right medial temporal region. Ictal SPECT (**b**): large right temporal hyperperfusion extended to the lateral temporal regions and to the left insula (axial left, sagittal right).

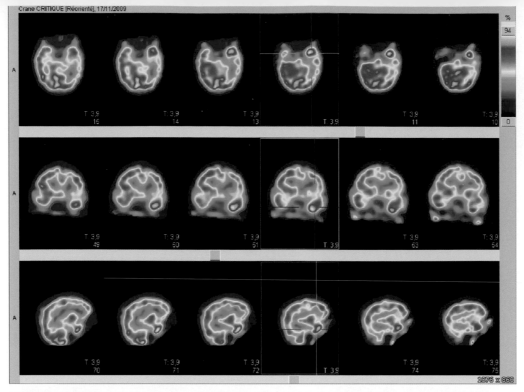

Fig. 20.4. Ictal SPECT: significant hyperperfusion of the left temporal pole and left anterior basal temporal region surrounded by a very large ipsilateral hypoperfusion.

(a)

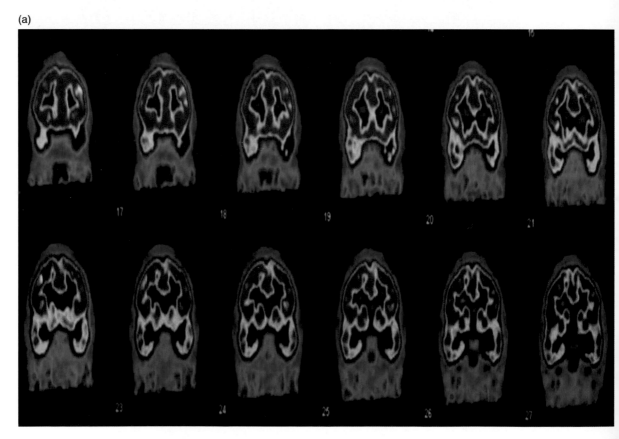

Fig. 20.5a.

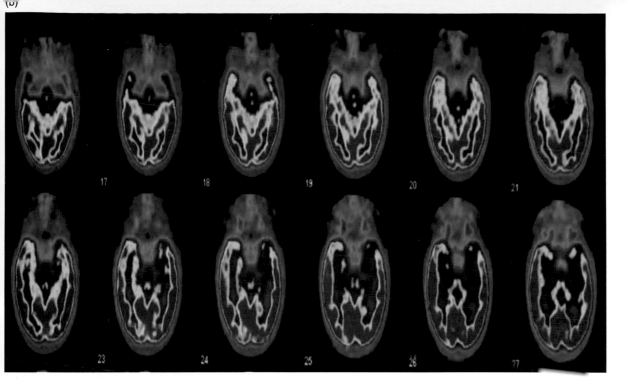

Fig. 20.5b. (*cont.*)

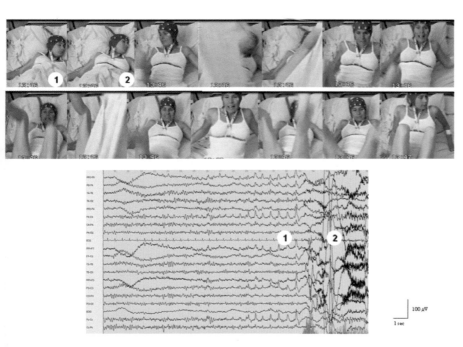

Fig. 22.1. Video-EEG recording: ictal EEG was characterized by initial high amplitude ictal Spikes, being of maximal amplitude on channels FP2, F8, F4, F2, FP1 (monopolar mortage, common average spikes).

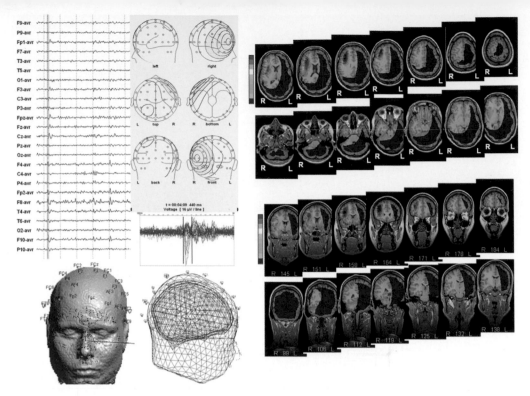

Fig. 22.2. High resolution EEG: Surface interictal spikes were recorded with 64 channels and a Hz sampling rate as well as amplitude cartography (using focus software).

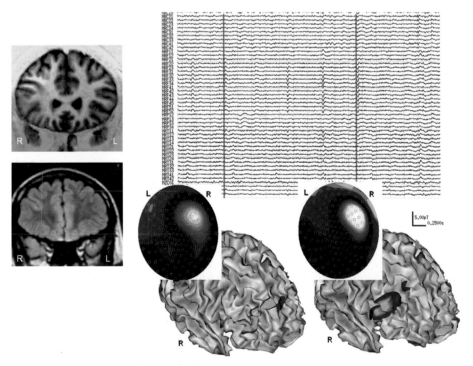

Fig. 22.3. A: Magnetoencephalography (MEG); B: MWG source localization; C: preoperative MRI.

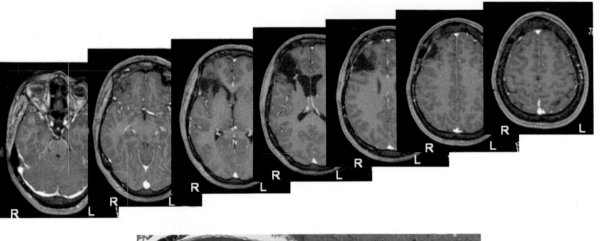

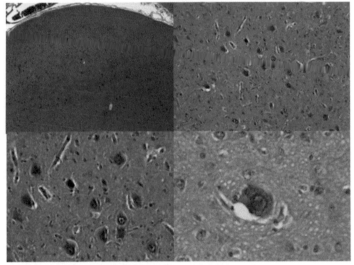

Fig. 22.4. Postoperative cerebral MRI (axial slices).

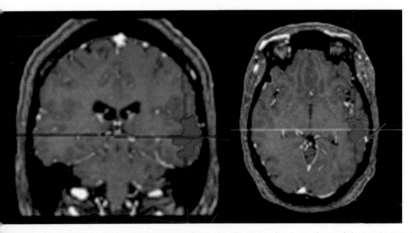

Fig. 24.4. MSI (MRI coregistered with MEG-dipole localisation): dipole analysis of the ictal MEG showed focal spike formation (red) in the left temporal region (infrasylvic, at the posterior portions of the superior and medial temporal gyri and posteriorly to the angular gyrus).

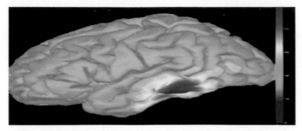

Fig. 24.5. The averaged dipole analysis (LORETA-analysis with interictal MEG) revealed a similar localization.

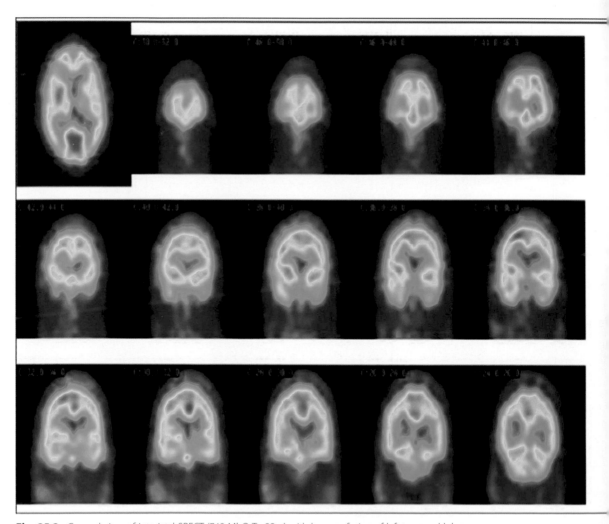

Fig. 25.2. Coronal view of interictal SPECT (740 MbQ-Tc-99m) with hypoperfusion of left temperal lobe.

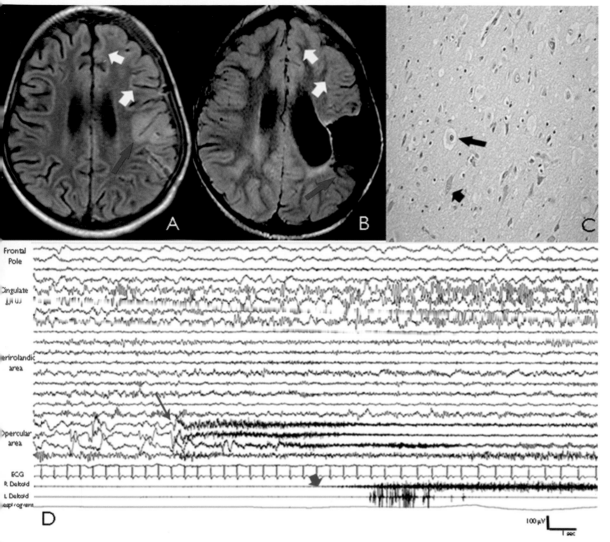

Fig. 37.1. MRI and EEG findings (**A**) Preoperative MRI (FLAIR). Abnormal gyral pattern, cortical thickness and blurring of the gray-white matter junction in the left frontal lobe (white arrows) and increased signal intensity in the left frontal operculum (red arrow). (**B**) Postoperative MRI (T1 weighted image). Abnormal gyral pattern, cortical thickness and blurring of the gray–white matter junction in the left frontal pole (white arrow) and postsurgical vacuum area (red arrow). (**C**) Histopathology. Hematoxylin and eosin staining of the paraffin-embedded surgical specimen clearly demonstrates the neuropathological hallmarks of FCD IIb, i.e. dysmorphic neurons (black arrowhead) and balloon cells (black arrow). (**D**) SEEG recordings showing interictal spikes and waves at the contacts exploring the left opercular area. At seizure onset (red arrow), the interictal abnormalities stop and low voltage fast activity occurs at the same contacts. Electromyographic recordings disclose a contraction of the right arm starting five seconds after the first EEG modification (red arrowhead).

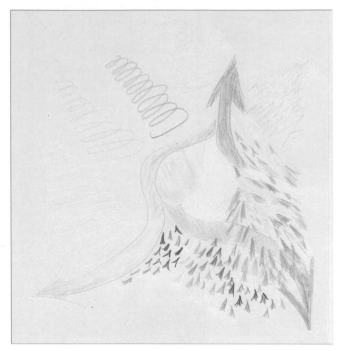

Fig. 29.3. Patient drawing of elementary-optic hallucination in hemianoptic field.

(a) (b)

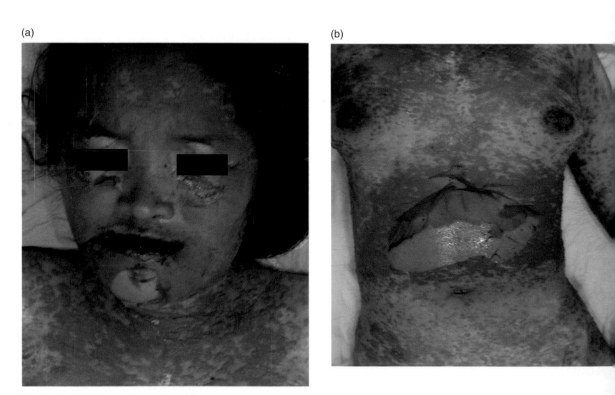

Fig. 50.1. Multiple maculopapule rashes.

Paraneoplastic limbic encephalitis

Barbara Schmalbach and Nicolas Lang

Clinical history

A 68-year-old male patient with a past medical history of arterial hypertension, alcohol and nicotine abuse was referred to our hospital because of acute-onset short-term memory loss with behavioral problems. Upon closer enquiry, the patient described episodes with a sense of an offensive smell followed by the sensation of chills with visible goose bumps. These episodes occurred approximately 10 20 times per day.

General history

Smoking, alcohol abuse, arterial hypertension.

Examination

On neurological examination the patient was disorientated in time and place, and to some extent in person. Neuropsychological testing mainly demonstrated deficits in phasic alertness and enhanced loss due to interference. Furthermore, testing of short-term memory and verbal working memory showed noticeable problems. Apart from that, there was no evidence for other neurological or psychiatric deficits.

Special studies

MRI of the brain showed bilateral mesio-temporal swelling (Fig. 1) without gadolinium uptake. Interictal surface EEG showed intermittent bilateral fronto-temporal slowing. Apart from that, frequent EEG seizures originating from the right and left temporal regions could be observed (Fig. 2). Cerebrospinal fluid (CSF) was negative except for a modest elevation in protein. Serum and CSF were negative for voltage-gated potassium channel (VGKC)- antibodies, onco-neural antibodies (anti-Hu, Ma, CV2), GAD anti-

bodies, but positive for voltage-gated calcium channel (VGCC)- antibodies (PQ-type).

Follow-up

An anti-inflammatory treatment with intravenous steroids (1000 mg methylprednisolone/day) for 5 days and an antiepileptic treatment (1000 mg levetiracetam/day) was initiated, which rendered the patient seizure free within 24 hours. Altered behavior and short-term memory loss were no longer detectable. In view of his significant smoking history, a paraneoplastic genesis was considered and a thoracic CT scan was arranged,

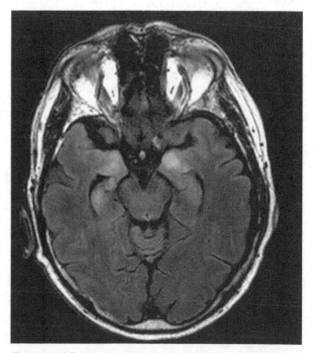

Fig. 1. Axial fluid-attenuated inversion recovery (FLAIR) images revealed hyperintense bilateral mesio-temporal edema.

Case Studies in Epilepsy, ed. Hermann Stefan, Elinor Ben-Menachem, Patrick Chauvel and Renzo Guerrini. Published by Cambridge University Press. © Hermann Stefan, Elinor Ben-Menachem, Patrick Chauvel and Renzo Guerrini 2012.

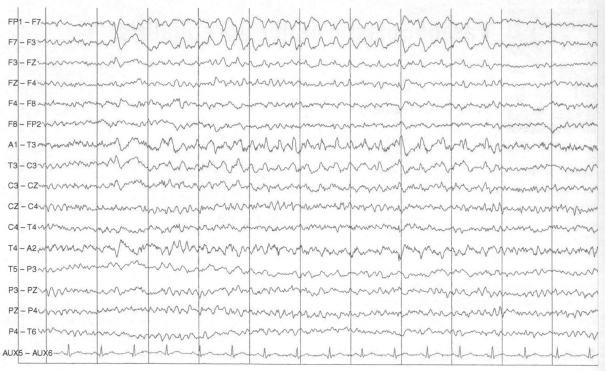

Fig. 2. Surface EEG demonstrated focal seizures originating from both temporal regions, here from the left.

which revealed a right hilary lymphadenopathy highly suggestive of bronchogenic carcinoma. Subsequent bronchoscopy with endosonography and transbronchial puncture verified right small cell lung carcinoma (SCLC) of the oat cell type in the stadium of limited disease. Furthermore, immunohistochemistry showed positive staining with CD56, chromogranin and synaptophysin. The patient received four cycles of a combined chemotherapy with cisplatin and etoposide, which led to a complete remission of the small cell lung carcinoma. A prophylactic cerebral radiation and thoracical radiation was planned, but had to be postponed due to aggravation of neurological symptoms, such as simple focal seizures, dizziness, and fatigue. The patient was once more treated with a pulse of methylprednisolone and levetiracetam combined with lorazepam, which ameliorated the symptoms of limbic encephalitis again.

Diagnosis

Limbic encephalitis presenting as a paraneoplastic manifestation of limited disease small cell lung cancer.

General remarks

Paraneoplastic limbic encephalitis (PLE) is defined as an inflammation of the anteromedial temporal cortex, hippocampus, and amygdale due to a misdirected tumor-activated antibody response that damages host neural tissue. This happens because antigens in the CNS resemble antigens found ectopically in malignancies, which trigger a protective immune response directed against CNS tissue.

Clinical hallmarks are anterograde memory impairment, temporal lobe seizures and psychiatric symptoms. In 60%–70% the neurologic symptoms precede the cancer diagnosis. The diagnostic procedure should include MRI, which typically shows characteristic non-enhancing signal changes in the mesial temporal lobes followed by atrophy at later stages, EEG with temporal epileptiform activity, and focal or diffuse slowing as well as cerebrospinal fluid examination, which may be normal or may show a modest elevation in protein and lymphocytic pleocytosis. The differential diagnoses include primary psychiatric illness, viral encephalitis, Creutzfeld–Jakob disease (CJD), vasculitis, herpes simplex, encephalitis, and non-paraneoplastic autoimmune encephalitis.

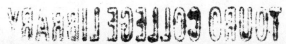 TOURO COLLEGE LIBRARY

Once limbic encephalitis has been diagnosed a thorough search for malignancy must be conducted with thoracical and abdominal CT scan, gynecologic examination including mammography, urologic examination, or even fluorodeoxyglucose positron emission tomography of the whole body (FDG-PET) having in mind typical malignancies associated with PLE: small cell lung carcinoma (SCLC), which is the most common tumor associated with PLE, testicular cancer, other types of lung cancer, breast cancer, lymphoma, thymoma, ovarian teratoma, adenocarcinoma of the colon, and esophageal carcinoma.

Several autoantibodies are associated with PLE. They can generally be divided into two main classes: the classical onconeuronal antibodies that are directed against intracellular antigens (anti-Hu-, anti-Ma2-, anti-CV2/CRMP5-, anti-Ri-, and anti-amphiphysin-antibodies) and antibodies directed against surface proteins, which may also be associated with a non-paraneoplastic form of limbic encephalitis (anti-VGKC complex-, anti-NMDAR-, anti-AMPAR-, and anti-GABA(b)R antibodies). However, it should be noted that, although autoantibody findings may be useful regarding etiology and prognosis, up to 30% of patients with PLE and cancer have negative antibody studies. If initial evaluation for malignancy is negative, it should be repeated after a few months.

Treatment includes eradication of the underlying malignancy, which leads to a removal of antigen source and suppression of the immune reaction with corticosteroids or ivIg optionally also with plasma exchange or immune apheresis. A more extensive immunosuppression with cyclophosphamide, mycophenolate mofetil, and with antibodies such as rituximab is considerable in selected cases. However, response to immunosuppressive therapy is poor in PLE associated with classical onconeuronal antibodies, whereas PLE associated with surface antibodies shows a much better therapeutic response.

Special remarks

The classical concept of limbic encephalitis has changed recently: patients with a non-paraneoplastic form of limbic encephalitis have increasingly been recognized. In these patients without an underlying malignancy, antibodies against surface proteins were detected, among them antibodies against the VGKC complex, NMDAR, AMPAR, GABAR and GAD. Response to immunotherapy is markedly better in these non-paraneoplastic forms.

Suggested reading

Foster AR, Caplan JP. Paraneoplastic limbic encephalitis. *Psychosomatics* 2009; **50**: 108–13.

Grisold W, Giometto B, Vitaliani R, Obesndorfer S. Current approaches to the treatment of paraneoplastic encephalitis. *Ther Adv Neurol Disord* 2011; **4**: 237–48.

Vernino S, Geschwind M, Boeve B. Autoimmune encephalitis. *Neurologist* 2007; **13**: 140–7.

Vincent A, Bien CG, Irani SR, Waters P. Autoantibodies associated with diseases of the CNS: new developments and future challenges. *Lancet Neurol* 2011; **10**: 759–72.

TOURO COLLEGE LIBRARY

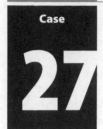

Case

27

Really a cerebrovascular story?

Burkhard Kasper and Hermann Stefan

Clinical history

A 60-year-old man came to the epilepsy outpatient unit for the first time, reporting about a 6–9 months' history of short episodic speech disturbances. He reported about the MRI finding of a subacute left hemispheric ischemia on an outside MRI weeks ago, the diagnosis of TIAs, and that none of the subsequent cardiovascular investigations including transesophageal echo and cardiac scintigram carried out so far had had any significant result. He then reported a dynamic progression of his symptoms, starting with rare and mild difficulties in finding words, e.g., while on the telephone, which had increased in frequency and strength during the last few weeks.

Examination

On examination, he had a mild, but permanent aphasic speech disturbance with semantic and phonematic paraphasias. He had developed mild headaches, had no nausea, vomiting, or any other focal neurological sign, but aphasia.

Special studies (Figs. 1, 2)

Detailed history revealed that, starting within the last month prior to the visit, he had developed new symptoms with an episodic warm feeling accompanied by slight tingling and numbness starting in perioral regions and spreading towards the upper right body quadrant. He also noted piloerection and flush in this area. Conciousness was never disturbed. EEG showed intermittent delta-slowing frontotemporal left without

spiking. MRI review showed left insular diffuse lesion with contrast enhancement. Actual MRI showed large ring-enhancing lesion with edema and mass effect.

Follow-up

AED treatment was able to improve seizure symptoms. The patient was treated with radiochemotherapy, then lost to further follow-up.

Diagnosis

Simple partial seizures with somatosensory and autonomous symptoms due to malignant primary brain neoplasm.

General remarks

New onset seizures in the higher age group is highly suspicious of an underlying neoplastic lesion, i.e., a primary tumor or metastasis. In this case episodic speech disturbances led to a diagnosis of TIAs and a contrast-enhancing MRI lesion was interpreted as subacute cortical infarction. Simple partial seizures developed within a few months, but remained unrecognized due to their unusual appearance. Progression of aphasic symptoms from subjectively episodic to an obvious permanent speech disturbance did not immediately lead to new investigations. Therefore, tumor diagnosis was made late in the course. The combination of seizures plus a progressing neurological deficit should point to a malignant cause.

Suggested reading

Le Blanc FE, Rasmussen T. Cerebral seizures and brain tumors. In PI Vinken, GW Bruyn, eds. *Handbook of Clinical Neurology:*

The Epilepsies. Amsterdam: Elsevier, 1974, vol 15, 295–301.

Moots PL. Pitfalls in the management of patients with malignant gliomas. *Semin Neurol* 1998; 18: 257–65.

Moots PL, Maciunas RJ, Eisert DR, et al. The course of seizure disorders in patients with malignant gliomas. *Arch Neurol* 1995; 52: 717–24.

Case Studies in Epilepsy, ed. Hermann Stefan, Elinor Ben-Menachem, Patrick Chauvel and Renzo Guerrini. Published by Cambridge University Press. © Hermann Stefan, Elinor Ben-Menachem, Patrick Chauvel and Renzo Guerrini 2012.

TOURO COLLEGE LIBRARY

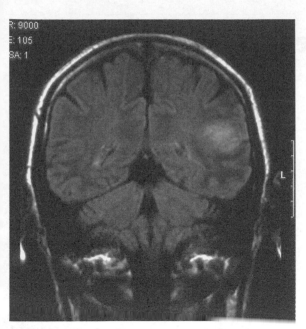

Fig. 1. First MRI.

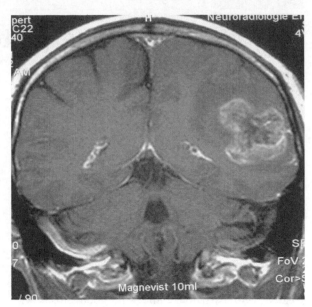

Fig. 2. Follow-up MRI.

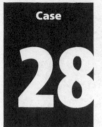
28 Sudden unexpected death in epilepsy – the ultimate failure

Elinor Ben-Menachem

This man was born in 1973. At the age of 12 he was involved in a traffic accident and received a left frontotemporal fracture as well as an orbital fracture and left-sided oculomotorius paresis. The most recent MRI showed left-sided frontal lobe defects as seen in an old traumatic brain injury. Shortly thereafter he developed focal onset epilepsy with frequent generalized tonic–clonic seizures. He was treated with carbamazepine with good effect, with sporadic seizures often when he forgot to take his medication.

During the years of 2000–2003 he had three episodes of focal status epilepticus. He was then started on levetiracetam and he never had status epilepticus again. Besides levetiracetam, he was taking phenytoin and valproate, which he had done for many years. His medication was not changed after starting levetiracetam, since he was essentially seizure free without side effects after then. The only time he had seizures after 2003 was when he had drunk alcohol or forgotten his tablets, which occurred two or three times a year.

When he was 33 years old, he finally moved out of his family home and got himself his own apartment. He had a stable job at a music store and enjoyed his work and his social life with his friends, but it was hard to convince him not to drink alcohol at parties. His parents and sister often called him and checked up on him. When he didn't answer the phone one morning in January 2008, they rushed to his apartment and found him face down in bed with his pyjamas on. The autopsy did not find any reason for his death and he did not have alcohol in his blood. The diagnosis after autopsy was sudden unexpected death in epilepsy or SUDEP.

Lesson learned

The definition of SUDEP is "sudden, unexpected, witnessed or unwitnessed, non-traumatic and non-drowning death in a patient with epilepsy where the postmortem examination does not reveal a toxicologic or anatomic cause of death, with or without evidence of a seizure and excluding documented status epilepticus" (Nashef and Brown, 1996).

The risk factors associated with SUDEP are (1) a history of generalized tonic–clonic seizures; (2) high number of GTCS; (3) frequent occurrence of seizures; (4) subtherapeutic AED levels (often due to noncompliance); (5) young adults, but seldom children; (6) a long history of epilepsy; (7) early onset of epilepsy; (8) antiepileptic drug polytherapy; (9) frequent changes in antiepileptic drugs; and (10) IQ under 70 (Langan et al., 2005; Tellez-Zenteno et al., 2005; Tomson et al., 2005).

In other words, SUDEP is not rare among patients with uncontrolled epilepsy. Risk of SUDEP is nearly four times greater in persons with 3 to 12 GTCS per year than in persons with 0 to 2 GTCS per year (Nilsson et al., 1999). Our patient actually had six of the risk factors described above: (a) history of generalized seizures and even status epilepticus; (b) seizures that re-occurred, albeit because of external factors, but he was not seizure free; (c) subtherapeutic AED levels because of noncompliance; (d) young adult; (e) early onset of epilepsy at the age of 12; and (f) polytherapy with antiepileptic drugs since he was taking three at the time of death. I would personally like to add another risk factor that I think is important, but is not mentioned in the literature and that is living alone. Most of my patients that have died in SUDEP were those living alone or were alone most of the time, especially at night.

Case Studies in Epilepsy, ed. Hermann Stefan, Elinor Ben-Menachem, Patrick Chauvel and Renzo Guerrini. Published by Cambridge University Press. © Hermann Stefan, Elinor Ben-Menachem, Patrick Chauvel and Renzo Guerrini 2012.

So, the main lesson in this case is that SUDEP is not rare among patients with uncontrolled epilepsy, especially young adults. Patients at risk should be identified and they and their families educated. It is important to stress risk factors that are controllable, such as compliance, and the importance of controlling alcohol consumption so as not to exacerbate seizures. The physician should try to work with the patient to control seizures, especially generalized tonic–clonic seizures as best as possible. In other words, optimize seizure control as promptly as possible. Re-evaluate epilepsy diagnosis and treatment as soon as two AEDs have failed. Consider epilepsy surgery at that point and maximize compliance with AEDs (So, 2008).

Even for patients with new-onset epilepsy, the idea of compliance should be stressed in order to decrease the risk of repeated seizures and possible SUDEP. Many relatives say that they wished they had been forewarned about the existence of SUDEP. There are many websites such as epilepsy.com as well as printed information, which discuss SUDEP as a part of the general education on epilepsy. This may be a more palatable way of introducing the subject to new onset patients who will be receiving antiepileptic drugs for the first time.

Suggested reading

Langan Y, Nashef L, Sander JW. Case-control study of SUDEP. *Neurology* 2005; **64**: 1131–3.

Nashef L, Brown S. Epilepsy and sudden death. *Lancet* 1996; **348**: 1324–5.

Nilsson L, Farahmand BY, Persson PG, Thiblin I, Tomson T. Risk factors for sudden unexpected death in epilepsy: a case-control study. *Lancet* 1999; **353**: 888–93.

So E. What is known about the mechanisms underlying SUDEP, *Epilepsia* 2008; **49**: 93–8.

Tellez-Zenteno JF, Ronquillo LH, Wiebe S. Sudden unexpected death in epilepsy: evidence-based analysis of incidence and risk factors. *Epilepsy Res* 2005; **65**: 101–15.

Tomson T, Walczak T, Sillanpaa M, Sander JW. Sudden unexpected death in epilepsy: a review of incidence and risk factors. *Epilepsia* 2005; **46**: 54–61.

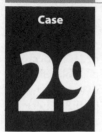

Case 29

Blind but able to see

Burkhard Kasper and Hermann Stefan

Clinical history

A 51-year old female was referred from a general hospital due to a series of tonic–clonic seizures during a febrile viral infection. In the past she had already experienced a few tonic–clonic seizures related to recurrent small hemorrhages from a left parieto-occipital cavernoma. A previous attempt to remove this lesion had failed, thereby causing a permanent deficit of dyschromatopsia and prosopagnosia. However, seizures had not recurred under AED therapy up to now. After acute treatment of generalized seizures, she first complained of total blindness and afterwards of permanent difficulties with reading or watching TV. Simultaneously with severe visual complaints, she very excitedly reported having regained her ability to see colors and faces (Fig. 1).

Examination

On first acute examination she showed no visual responses to external stimuli and was unable to recognize things held in front of her eyes, but recognized some by touching them with her hands. She appeared fully awake, unless some complex partial seizures seemed to interrupt at this stage. After cessation of recognizable seizures by treatment, she had obvious permanent hemianopsia to the right. During the next days, detailed questioning revealed the description of intense colorful perceptions in the blind hemifield, accompanied by visuoscenic experiences including faces related to her daily life at home (Fig. 2).

Special studies

In the stage of cortical blindness, acute imaging with CT and MRI including non-invasive angiography and cerebrospinal fluid investigation ruled out a new bleed, infarction or inflammatory cause. Video–EEG was established 1 day later, when she reported "being able to see again, but limited" due to hemianopsia, abundant focal seizure patterns restricted to occipital lobe electrodes were detected (Fig. 3).

Follow-up

Hemianopsia and visual-optic elementary and complex hallucinations persisted for 1 week. While 3000 mg levetiracetam were not able to end this, vision improved and hallucinations vanished after introduction of 200 mg lacosamide adding on a topiramate therapy. However, a striking right monocular visual field restriction still persisted up to discharge from our hospital.

Diagnosis

Ictal cortical blindness, hemianopsia, and complex visual hallucinations due to cavernoma-related occipital lobe epilepsy.

General remarks

Elementary sensory hallucinations are fascinating symptoms, closely related to focal epileptic discharges and therefore bear highly localizing value. In this patient, severe loss of function with transient blindness leading to 1-week hemianopsia was combined with a nearly continous experience of optic sensation, both elementary and complex scenic. The patient was fascinated, excited, and very pleased about the latter, because these seizure symptoms in her view "re-installed" her ability to clearly differentiate colors and recognize faces, which was lost due to the iatrogenic occipital lesioning. All her symptoms were clearly related to ongoing occipital seizure activity only.

Case Studies in Epilepsy, ed. Hermann Stefan, Elinor Ben-Menachem, Patrick Chauvel and Renzo Guerrini. Published by Cambridge University Press. © Hermann Stefan, Elinor Ben-Menachem, Patrick Chauvel and Renzo Guerrini 2012.

(a)

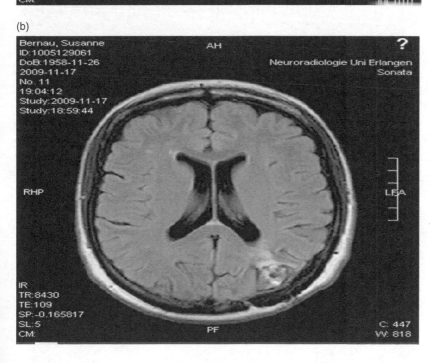

(b)

Fig. 1(a) and (b). MRI showing left occipital cavernoma and iatrogenic defect superior to it

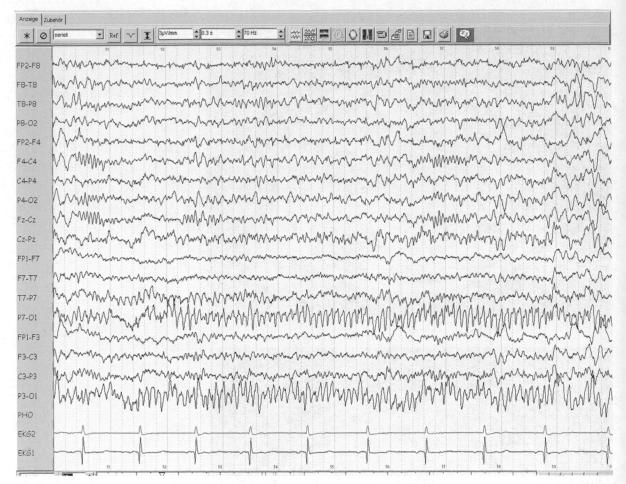

Fig. 2. EEG displaying ongoing rhythmic epileptic activity in occipital region (P7-O1, P3-O1).

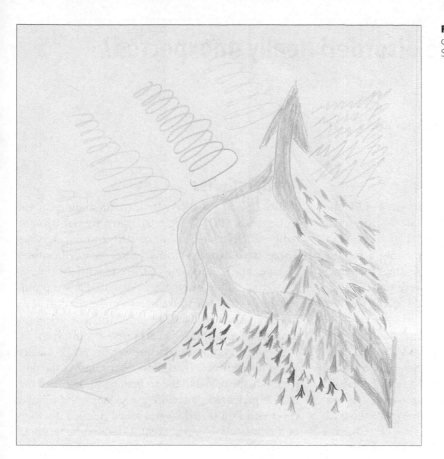

Fig. 3. Patient drawing of elementary-optic hallucination in hemianoptic field. See color plate section.

Suggested reading

Salanova V, Andermann F, Olivier A, Rasmussen T, Quesney LF. Occipital lobe epilepsy: electroclinical manifestations, electrocorticography, cortical stimulation and outcome in 42 patients treated between 1930 and 1991. Surgery of occipital lobe epilepsy. *Brain* 1992; **115**: 1655–80.

Williamson PD, Thadani VM, Darcey TM, *et al.* Occipital lobe epilepsy: clinical characteristics, seizure spread patterns, and results of surgery. *Ann Neurol* 1992; **31**: 3–13.

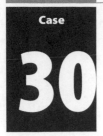

Case

30

Seizure disorder! Really unexpected?

Burkhard Kasper and Hermann Stefan

Clinical history

A 26-year-old female was sent for video–EEG for verification of suspected psychogenic non-epileptic seizures, which were highly suggested by her general neurologist. Attacks were noted beginning 9 months before her hospital visit, with increasing frequency up to once per day. These attacks were noticed from the awake state only and described quite vaguely. The patient always emphasized not to have *any* clue for the presence of a disorder, only others would repeatedly report that something was wrong with her from time to time. The mother and a friend reported about episodes of slight disorientation, reduced responses, shivering-like movements, and mainly incoherent talking. Her neurologist witnessed such an attack once while talking to her about a traumatic experience – she had been the victim of a sexual crime some years ago. The patient herself reported to believe the attacks were triggered by emotional stimuli, e.g., conflict situations at home. Furthermore, she had a history of a major depressive episode in the previous year with a suicide attempt and alcohol misuse and also some symptoms of self-injuring behavior.

Examination

Psychopathologically, she had mild symptoms of reduced affect only. Arms and hands showed old and subacute small skin wounds from scratching (earlier she had used tinned-food lids to cut herself). Neurologically, mild spastic hemisymptoms were found with brisk reflexes on the left arm and leg; in addition, she reported about surgical correction of a pes equinus in childhood.

Special studies

Video–EEG revealed very frequent monomorphic epileptic spikes (Fig. 1), detected 100% by right frontotemporal electrodes in awake state and during sleep. Three unequivocal seizures were recorded without precipitating factors, one of them from sleep (Fig. 2). The latter did not display any recognizable symptoms, but she failed to remember a test word given during the EEG pattern. One seizure while on the telephone showed interruption of conciousness with arrest and hypomotor symptoms. A third seizure while inactive was unrecognizable by clinical means, but in the post-ictal state she talked to the woman beside her, as if they had experienced something together. She recalled experiences quite vividly and asked detailed questions as if talking about a real event. Later on, she was completely amnesic about this. Psychogenic attacks were not seen. She performed normally in neuropsychological test batteries. Cranial MRI showed a complex congenital malformation of cortical development with a right predominant frontotemporal-perisylvian schizencephaly–polymicrogyria complex (Fig. 3).

Follow-up

Video–EEG was demonstrated to the patient and relatives, thereby confirming the patient's amnesia for the episodes and approving similarity to observations at home. A treatment with lamotrigine was initiated.

Diagnosis

Symptomatic partial epilepsy with complex partial seizures caused by congenital CNS malformation.

Case Studies in Epilepsy, ed. Hermann Stefan, Elinor Ben-Menachem, Patrick Chauvel and Renzo Guerrini. Published by Cambridge University Press. © Hermann Stefan, Elinor Ben-Menachem, Patrick Chauvel and Renzo Guerrini 2012.

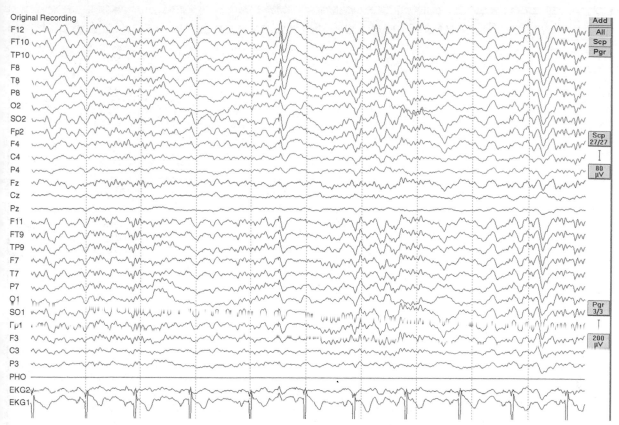

Fig. 1. Interictal spikes right frontotemporal.

General remarks

Psychogenic non-epileptic seizures (PNESs) often are embedded into a scenario of psychiatric comorbidity such as depression, post-traumatic stress disorder, or personality disorder. PNESs tend to be described with striking, often prolonged, motor symptoms, or fainting-like, or with rather vague symptoms with presumed impairment of conciousness. Emotional and psychic triggers are common. PNESs usually do not arise from sleep. Not untypically, a remote traumatic experience, e.g., rape,

severe accident, or a loved one's death, is revealed by history taking. Comorbid "true" seizures might be present. However, as illustrated above, even a full risk scenario suggesting PNES is no reliable indicator of this diagnosis. A neurological deficit is unusual in patients with isolated PNESs. Many forms of epileptic seizures can be mistaken for PNES due to their mild, vague or bizarre semiology. Video–EEG at a referral center is the gold-standard for differentiating PNES and epileptic seizures.

Suggested reading

Wu YW, Lindan CE, Henning LH, *et al.* Neuroimaging abnormalities in infants with congenital hemiparesis. *Pediatr Neurol* 2006; **35**: 191–6.

Barkovich AJ, Kuzniecky RI, Jackson GD, Guerrini R, Dobyns WB. A developmental and genetic classification for malformations of cortical development. *Neurology* 2005; **65**: 1873–87.

Bodde NM, Brooks JL, Baker GA, *et al.* Psychogenic non-epileptic seizures – definition, etiology, treatment and prognostic issues: a critical review. *Seizure* 2009; **18**: 543–53.

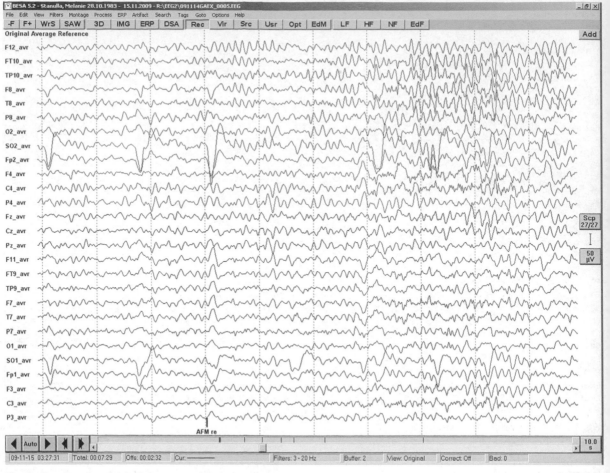

Fig. 2. Development of right frontotemporal ictal pattern.

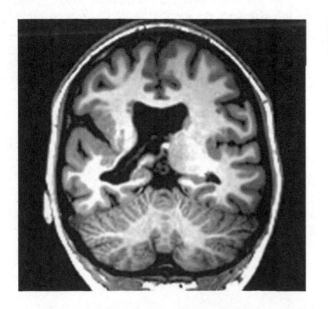

Fig. 3. Coronary T1 image showing complex congenital malformation with right schizencephaly-polymicrogyria complex, milder left perisylvian polymicrogyria and absent septum.

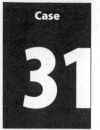

Transient epileptic amnesia in late onset epilepsy

Elisabeth Pauli and Hermann Stefan

Clinical history

A 59-year-old male school Principal was referred from a psychiatric hospital to the epilepsy outpatient unit. One year ago he had suddenly developed striking behavioral abnormalities. His wife noticed acute lapses of memory and mental black-outs. She described idiosyncratic episodic behavioral disturbances, in which he gesticulated strangely. When involved in talks, he answered inadequately, lacking meaning. In conferences, he seemed confused, jumping from theme to theme, demonstrating mental leaps. Initially, he himself did not notice these incidents, but complained about feeling under par, about headaches, and sleep disturbances. Finally, he and his wife took notice of a progression of his symptoms, with increasing memory disturbances, episodes of word finding deficits, and most disturbingly, loss of memory for whole episodes. For example, he and colleagues attended a 3-day-conference in another city, where he gave a lecture and received a prize. But afterwards the complete episode – including his lecturing – was erased from his memory. Similar events occurred over the following months: he could not remember a short vacation trip with his family at New Year. And, most wearing, he lost most memories from a 4-week overseas trip, where he accompanied a graduating student exchange.

Finally, he consulted a neurologist, who referred him to psychiatry with the suspicion of dementia and panic disorder. There, a mild cognitive impairment was diagnosed. In the course of the stay the psychiatrist witnessed symptoms with gesticulation and strange reactions. He suspected a complex partial seizure and referred him to the epilepsy unit.

Examination

Video–EEG monitoring showed no epileptiform transients, no seizure patterns. But ictal recordings showed many epileptic events, clinically stereotypical, but differing in duration and intensity. The shortest consisted of tachycardia only, with frequencies up to 180 bpm. In the case of longer duration, semiology emerged with a peculiar facial expression, distortion, and opening of the mouth, sighing, uttering "yes, yes, yes," and agitation with both hands. Then symptomatology passed into swaying the upper parts of the body, accompanied by an ecstatic facial expression. The clouding of consciousness seemed only mild, the patient gave correct answers, and he could repeat spoken words and was able to read. However, subsequently he was completely amnesic about the whole event.

Special studies

The MRI did not detect a structural lesion, while ictal SPECT demonstrated focal enhanced perfusion in the left anterior temporal lobe. Neuropsychological evaluation revealed a moderate impairment of anterograde verbal memory functions and mild depression.

Follow-up

AED treatment did improve seizure symptoms. After titration, he became seizure free. Neuropsychological recovery was observed with verbal memory returned to the normal range and improvement of depression.

Diagnosis

Temporal lobe epilepsy.

Case Studies in Epilepsy, ed. Hermann Stefan, Elinor Ben-Menachem, Patrick Chauvel and Renzo Guerrini. Published by Cambridge University Press. © Hermann Stefan, Elinor Ben-Menachem, Patrick Chauvel and Renzo Guerrini 2012.

General remarks

Memory impairment with loss of episodic memories only from selected events is usually interpreted as psychogenic, or as an indication of dementia. However, episodic memory deficits, transient amnesia, and accelerated forgetting are also described in epilepsy patients. Not rarely, epilepsy patients complain about lacking memories of remote events or even about forgetting whole episodes only weeks or months ago; sometimes their memories are faded or blurred, sometimes completely erased.

Suggested reading

Butler CR, Zeman AZ. Recent insight into the impairment of memory in epilepsy: transient epileptic amnesia, accelerated long-term forgetting and remote memory impairment. *Brain* 2008; **131**: 2243–63.

A really unexpected injury?

32

Wolfgang Graf and Hermann Stefan

Clinical history

A 36-year-old male patient was admitted to our epilepsy center for presurgical evaluations. During video–EEG assessment and drug withdrawal, several habitual complex partial seizures occurred, one of them with rapid secondary generalization. During the intense tonic phase of this generalized seizure – without any external trauma – a loud noise was noticeable indicating bone fracture. Afterwards, the patient complained about severe pain within his left upper arm.

General history

Seizures had started at 32 years of age. His epilepsy was classified as non-lesional with complex partial and secondary generalized seizures. Previously, treatment had included only three antiepileptic drugs (i.e., carbamazepine, lamotrigine, levetiracetam). No other relevant diseases existed. In particular, there was no evidence for previous fractures, osteopathy, or bone-specific symptoms such as ostalgia or bone malpositions.

Physical examination

Apparently, the patient kept his left upper arm in a relieving posture. Mobility of left upper arm was clearly reduced, even slight movements or local pressure were extremely painful. Beyond that, the neurological examination was completely normal.

Special studies

X-ray showed a displaced fracture of the left humeral head (Fig. 1(a)). Bone mineral density (BMD) of the lumbar spinal column and the femoral neck was measured by dual-energy X-ray absorptiometry (DEXA). The patient's DEXA measurement of femoral neck (Fig. 2) showed marginal pathologic BMD z-score (z-score = – 1), reflecting a reduced BMD of 1 standard deviation compared to the age- and sex-related reference population. BMD T-score was within the normal range. The lumbar spinal DEXA measurement was normal. Serum analysis revealed a low vitamin D3-level of 13.0 ng/ml (normal range 30.0 – 70.0 ng/ml) and normal calcium level.

Follow-up

After surgical treatment (Fig. 2) fracture healing proceeded without any complications. Under physical therapy in the post acute phase the patient reached an almost normal function and painless mobility of his left upper arm.

Imaging

Diagnosis

Humerus fracture due to a secondary generalized tonic–clonic seizure.

Discussion

Epilepsy patients face an increased fracture risk compared with the normal population. Preferred fracture localizations are the spinal column, ribs, and hip. The etiology of this increased fracture disposition in epilepsy patients is multifactorial. A significant part of epileptic seizures go along with falls and consecutive direct traumatic fractures. In addition, but under-recognized, muscular tension during seizures can be strong enough to induce a fracture, as shown here. Besides the risk factors of

Case Studies in Epilepsy, ed. Hermann Stefan, Elinor Ben-Menachem, Patrick Chauvel and Renzo Guerrini. Published by Cambridge University Press. © Hermann Stefan, Elinor Ben-Menachem, Patrick Chauvel and Renzo Guerrini 2012.

(a)

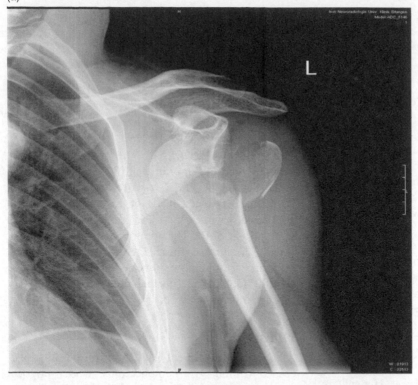

(b)

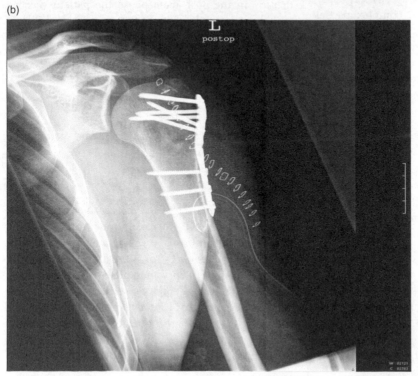

Fig. 1. Displaced fracture of the left proximal humerus emerging from the tonic phase of a secondary generalized tonic–clonic seizure without any external trauma before (a) and after surgical treatment (b) [source: Erlangen University Hospital, Dept. of Neuroradiology, Prof. A Dörfler].

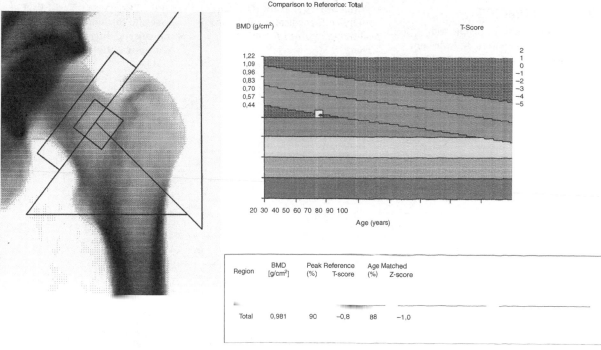

Fig. 2. DEXA-measurement of femoral neck. BMD Z-score (Z-score $= -1$) is marginal pathologic and reflects a reduced BMD compared to the age- and sex-related reference population, BMD T-score is within the normal range (Z-score $= -0.8$). [source: Erlangen University Hospital, Dept. of Internal Medicine 1, Division of Endocrinology and Diabetology, Prof. IA Harsch].

age-related osteoporosis or other pre-existing diseases, continuous treatment with antiepileptic drugs (AEDs) can have unfavorable effects on bone health. The postulated mechanisms of AED-related changes in bone metabolism are numerous. A main explanation seems to lie in increased vitamin D catabolism. Enzyme-inducing AEDs such as phenytoin (PHT), carbamazepine (CBZ), or phenobarbital (PB) induce p450 cytochromes, thereby increasing the hepatic turnover of vitamin D-metabolites (25-hydroxyvitamin D, 25-OHD). This results in lack of vitamin D, decreased calcium absorption, secondary hyperparathyroidism, increased calcium mobilization from the bone, and decreased bone mineral density (BMD) as well as osteomalacia. Similar effects on vitamin D metabolism have also been described for second-generation AEDs (e.g., valproic acid). Beyond that, several AEDs seem to have a direct negative effect on bone cells, bone turnover, and bone quality. Other influences on renal, intestinal, and hormonal functions with negative effects on bone health are known.

As a practical consequence, bone health in epilepsy patients should be carefully considered and monitored in order to identify and treat patients at risk. Dual-energy X-ray absorptiometry (DEXA) of lumbar spine and femoral neck is useful as the standard method for determination of BMD. BMD appears as the best predictor of fracture risk and the most valuable parameter to describe bone status. Biomarkers such as vitamin D and calcium levels give additional information about patients' bone health.

Four key notes seem mandatory in counseling:

1. The possible risks for bone health related to AED intake.
2. Information on how to positively influence bone health (e.g., adjustment of eating habits, physical activity, sun exposition, avoidance of falls).
3. Appropriate diagnostics and early substitution of vitamin D and calcium in case of significant risk.
4. Information about seizure-related injury risks including fractures during in-hospital video–EEG diagnostics.

Suggested reading

Pack A. Bone health in people with epilepsy: is it impaired and what are the risk factors? *Seizure* 2008; **17**: 181–6.

Petty SJ, O'Brien TJ, Wark JD, *et al.* Antiepileptic medication and bone health. *Osteoporos Int* 2007; **18**: 129–42.

Verrotti A, Coppola G, Parisi P, *et al.* Bone and calcium metabolism and antiepileptic drugs. *Clin Neurol Neurosurg* 2010; **112**: 1–10.

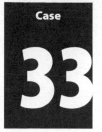

Epileptic negative myoclonus in benign rolandic epilepsy

Francesco Zellini and Renzo Guerrini

Clinical history

A 4½-year-old girl with normal psychomotor development was admitted to our hospital for abrupt onset of a coarse tremor and jerking of the right hand. The abnormal movements were arrhythmic and only obvious during skilled movements.

Tremor episodes started 3 days before admission with a daily frequency. They were spontaneously at rest or during actions and had a duration of a few seconds, without consciousness impairment

Family history

There was no family history of neuropsychiatric conditions.

Neurological examination

When the child was asked to maintain her arms outstretched, her right hand or the whole right arm exhibited repeated brief lapses. No other neurological signs were noticed.

Special studies

Polygraphic video–EEG recording revealed repetitive epileptic left centro-temporal sharp waves that were greatly enhanced during sleep At rest, these discharges were apparently infraclinic, but when the girl was asked to outstretch her arms, it became obvious that postural lapses of her right hand and arm were accompanied by a muscle silent period on the EMG channel sampling from the right arm muscles and by a time-locked sharp wave over the contralateral central region (see Fig. 1). This electroclinical pattern was typical of focal epileptic negative myoclonus. Brain MRI was normal.

Follow-up

Ethosuximide therapy was introduced, leading to a marked reduction of epileptic negative myoclonus episodes, which was paralleled by abatement of EEG discharges. Five months later a seemingly generalized seizure appeared during sleep. Valproate therapy was introduced while ethosuximide was discontinued, but negative myoclonus reappeared within a few days. Add-on clobazam treatment again controlled negative myoclonus and abated EEG discharges. The girl has now been seizure free for 1 year and her EEG has remained normal after clobazam discontinuation.

Diagnosis

Benign rolandic epilepsy with epileptic negative myoclonus (ENM).

General remarks

Benign childhood epilepsy with centro-temporal spikes or benign rolandic epilepsy (BRE) is the most common and characteristic form of "idiopathic" focal epilepsy, accounting for 16% of the epilepsies beginning before 15 years of age. The syndrome is characterize by: (1) onset between the ages of 2 and 13 with a peak around school age; (2) absence of neurologic or intellectual deficit; (3) focal seizures with motor signs, frequently associated with somatosensory symptoms and precipitated by sleep; (4) a spike focus located in the centro-temporal (rolandic) area with normal background EEG activity; (5) spontaneous remission during adolescence. Rolandic seizures involve one side of the face and the oropharyngeal muscles, comprising guttural sounds, contraction of the jaws, dysarthria, and

---

Case Studies in Epilepsy, ed. Hermann Stefan, Elinor Ben-Menachem, Patrick Chauvel and Renzo Guerrini. Published by Cambridge University Press. © Hermann Stefan, Elinor Ben-Menachem, Patrick Chauvel and Renzo Guerrini 2012.

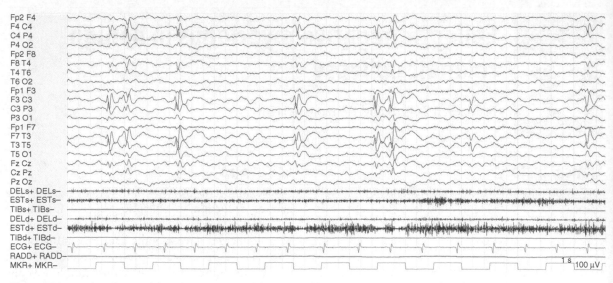

Fig. 1. EEG recording showing bilateral centro-temporal sharp waves that are more prominent on the left. The patient is keeping her upper limbs outstretched. Brief lapses of posture are captured on the right wrist extensor as brief pauses of ongoing EMG activity that are time locked to contralateral sharp and slow-wave complexes. Figure legend: DELs: Left deltoid; ESTs: Left wrist extensor; TIBs: Left tibialis anterior; DELd: Right deltoid; ESTd: Right wrist extensor; TIBd: right tibialis anterior.

profuse drooling of saliva. Interictal EEG abnormalities are an essential part of the syndrome. They are typically localized to the centro-temporal region, exhibiting a characteristic waveform, field of distribution, and activation by sleep. In a limited number of patients with benign rolandic epilepsy epileptic negative myoclonus may appear for a variable length of time. Neurophysiological studies have demonstrated that the muscle silent periods of epileptic negative myoclonus are accompanied by a rolandic waveform whose morphology is slightly different from that observed in the majority of patients, often with a prominent slow wave component Such waveform may predispose patients to seizure aggravation when carbamazepine is used. Complex genetic factors are thought to play a role in the pathogenesis of BRE, but the mechanisms at play are obscure. Seizures remit before the age of 16 in almost 100% of patients. The global prognosis of BRE, regarding social outcome and school achievement, appears as good as that for seizures. Considering the benign nature of the syndrome, any form of overtreatment should be avoided. A reasonable approach seems not to give any antiepileptic drug if no generalization of seizures occurs. There is no study demonstrating that treating rolandic epilepsy reduces the number of seizures and the overall outcome.

Special remarks

Negative myoclonus is an unspecific disorder that can be observed in a variety of physiological, as well as pathological conditions and is defined as "epileptic" if the jerking is related to brief pauses of ongoing EMG activity lastsing 50 to 400 ms that are time locked with contralateral spike-wave complexes over the central area. ENM can be observed in idiopathic, cryptogenic, and symptomatic epilepsies. Epileptic negative myoclonus in BRE is usually responsive to ethosuximide. Patients with BRE and epileptic negative myoclonus do not appear to have a different prognostic outlook with respect to those without ENM.

Future perspectives

In a benign condition such as epileptic negative myoclonus in BRE, the results of future clinical trials will doubtfully produce a relevant change in clinical practice. More important seems to be a precise recognition of an atypical form of BRE to avoid misdiagnosis, overtreatment, or even seizures aggravation.

Suggested reading

Fernandez-Torre JL, Otero B. Epileptic negative myoclonus in a case of atypical benign partial epilepsy of childhood: a detailed video-polygraphic study. *Seizure* 2004; **13**: 226–34.

Fujii A, Oguni H, Hirano Y, *et al.* Atypical benign partial epilepsy: recognition can prevent pseudocatastrophe. *Pediatr Neurol* 2010; **43**: 411–19.

Guerrini R, Dravet C, Genton P. Epileptic negative myoclonus. *Neurology* 1993; **43**: 1078–83.

Parmeggiani L, Seri S, Bonanni P. *et al.* Electrophysiological characterization of spontaneous and carbamazepine-induced epileptic negative myoclonus in benign childhood epilepsy with centro-temporal spikes. *Clin Neurophysiol* 2004; **115**:50–8.

Rubboli G, Tassinari CA. Negative myoclonus. An overview of its clinical features, pathophysiological mechanisms, and management. *Neurophysiol Clin* 2006; **36**: 337–43.

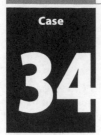

Case

34

Sporadic hemiplegic migraine

Francesco Zellini and Renzo Guerrini

Clinical history

A 17-year-old girl with normal psychomotor development was admitted to our hospital after developing a left hemiparesis that had progressed over 30 minutes and was followed by severe pulsating headache, referred to the right side of the head, with photophobia and drowsiness.

One year earlier, a previous episode had occurred, with transitory paresis and paresthesia involving the right side of the face and the right arm, followed by drowsiness, nausea, and vomit. MRI and MR angiography were reported as normal.

Family history

One cousin had migraine with visual aura.

Neurological examination

The patient exhibited left hemiparesis and drowsiness, with headache and nausea.

Special studies

EEG during the attack revealed continuous irregular delta activity over the right hemisphere (Fig. 1). Brain MRI was normal.

Follow-up

The patient recovered completely within 24 hours using analgesics. Verapamil therapy was started and no further episodes occurred in the following 2 years. Genetic testing revealed a *de novo* missense mutation in ATP1A2 gene.

Diagnosis

Sporadic hemiplegic migraine.

General remarks

Hemiplegic migraine is characterized by migraine with aura and reversible motor weakness.

Sporadic hemiplegic migraine is clinically similar to familial hemiplegic migraine (FHM). Both familial hemiplegic migraine and sporadic hemiplegic migraine are classified under migraine with aura in the *International Classification of Headache Disorders,* 2nd edn (ICHD-2). All attacks that meet the criteria for migraine and include reversible weakness (motor aura) lasting from 5 minutes to 24 hours should be coded as hemiplegic migraine (familial or sporadic) once other causes have been excluded.

Familial and sporadic hemiplegic migraine are genetically heterogenous. Mutations in three different genes, including *FHM-1* (*CACNA1A*) gene, the *FHM-2* (*ATP1A2*) gene, and the *FHM-3* (*SCN1A*) gene account for 50% to 70% of published families with familial hemiplegic migraine and are found in sporadic cases. Allelic to FHM are other channelopathies such as episodic ataxia and hypokalemic periodic paralysis.

The calcium channel blocker verapamil has been used effectively as a preventive and acute treatment for hemiplegic migraine. Other treatments reported to produce some benefit as preventive treatment of sporadic hemiplegic migraine include acetazolamide and patent foramen ovale closure in patients in whom migraine is associated with patent foramen ovale.

Special remarks

Transient hemiparesis with drowsiness and confusion, accompanied by unilateral slowing of EEG activity, could make the differential diagnosis between hemiplegic migraine attack and postictal weakness following a focal seizure difficult, especially in spor-

---

Case Studies in Epilepsy, ed. Hermann Stefan, Elinor Ben-Menachem, Patrick Chauvel and Renzo Guerrini. Published by Cambridge University Press. © Hermann Stefan, Elinor Ben-Menachem, Patrick Chauvel and Renzo Guerrini 2012.

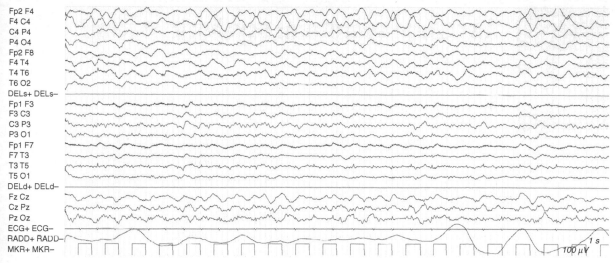

Fig. 1. EEG recording while the patient is awake shows asymmetric background activity with continuous high amplitude delta activity over the right hemisphere.

adic patients. Postictal headache is also frequent in patients with epilepsy A careful clinical history, and the progression of motor signs over 60, are more typical for hemiplegic migraine. A normal MRI is also necessary to exclude acute ischemic process or cerebral bleeding. The *ATP1A2* gene encodes for the α2 subunit of the Na, K-ATPase, hence suggesting a key role of cation trafficking in the pathophysiology of FHM. Most of the *ATP1A2* mutations are associated with pure hemiplegic migraine, without additional clinical symptoms. However, several FHM2 mutations have been associated with complications such as cerebellar ataxia, epilepsy, and mental retardation.

Verapamil was effective in our case as preventive therapy during the 2-year follow-up.

Future perspectives

The genetic basis of calcium channelopathies, including hemiplegic migraine, provides a unique opportunity to investigate their underlying mechanisms from the molecular to whole-organism levels. Studies of channelopathies may also lead to the identification of drugs for the treatment of genetically acquired channel disorders, as well as to novel therapeutic practices.

Suggested reading

Black DF. Sporadic and familial hemiplegic migraine: diagnosis and treatment. *Semin Neurol* 2006; **26**: 208–16.

de Vries B, Freilinger T, Vanmolkot KR, *et al.* Systematic analysis of three FHM genes in 39 sporadic patients with hemiplegic migraine. *Neurology* 2007; **69**: 2170–6.

International Headache Society Classification Subcommittee.

International Classification of Headache Disorders, 2nd edn. *Cephalalgia* 2004; **24**: 1–160.

Lastimosa AC. Treatment of sporadic hemiplegic migraine with calcium-channel blocker verapamil. *Neurology* 2003; **61**: 721–2.

Lemka M, Pienczk-Reclawowicz K, Pilarska E, *et al.* Cessation of sporadic hemiplegic migraine attacks after patent foramen ovale

closure. *Dev Med Child Neurol* 2009; **51**: 923–4.

Riant F, Ducros A, Ploton C, *et al.* De novo mutations in ATP1A2 and CACNA1A are frequent in early-onset sporadic hemiplegic migraine. *Neurology* 2010; **75**: 967–72.

Thomsen LL, Oestergaard E, Bjornsson A, *et al.* Screen for CACNA1A and ATP1A2 mutations in sporadic hemiplegic migraine patients. *Cephalalgia* 2008; **28**: 914–21.

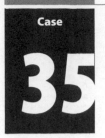

Case

35

A strange symptom: psychotic or ictal?

Burkhard Kasper and Hermann Stefan

Clinical history

A 35-year-old female had a history of major depression for several years. Then she developed episodes with a rather bizarre description of identity change. She reported about her experience to undergo a transformation of sexual identity towards male gender. This illusion affected her perception of herself and also her perception of other female persons nearby. These symptoms first-line were conceived as psychotic-hallucinatory symptoms within the context of her depression and antidepressant treatment before she visited a neurology department.

Examination

On examination, she was fully intact regarding neurological status; psychopathology was unremarkable with SSRI treatment.

Neurological scores
Special studies

Detailed history revealed a symptom sequence of an epigastric rising sensation accompanied by déjà-vu, which evolved into the complex delusional symptom of sexual change. Several times, further development to impaired conciousness was noted. Secondary generalization had never occurred. MRI revealed a foreign tissue lesion within the right amygdalar region, classified as ganglioglioma or dysembryoplastic neuroepithelial tumor. Video–EEG recording showed intermittent right temporal slowing with few epileptiform transients. Ictal recordings were not achieved (Figs. 1, 2).

Follow-up

So far, epilepsy surgery has not been performed, since her condition is stable with well-controlled epilepsy

with AED treatment. No progression has been observed on follow-up MRIs.

Diagnosis

Symptomatic partial epilepsy due to a tumorous lesion with psychic seizures and mood disorder.

General remarks

Psychiatric comorbidity is not rare in partial epilepsies. It may happen that the mood disorder precedes the manifestation of epilepsy by years. In this patient, the complex ictal psychic symptoms, represented by the delusion of sexual change, were not easily recognized by history taking as experiential phenomena related to seizure acitivity. Only when an obvious

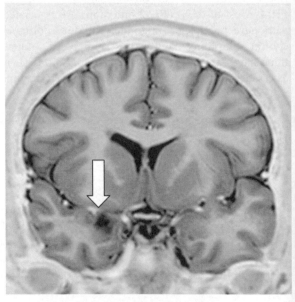

Fig. 1. MRI showing right amygdalar lesion.

Case Studies in Epilepsy, ed. Hermann Stefan, Elinor Ben-Menachem, Patrick Chauvel and Renzo Guerrini. Published by Cambridge University Press. © Hermann Stefan, Elinor Ben-Menachem, Patrick Chauvel and Renzo Guerrini 2012.

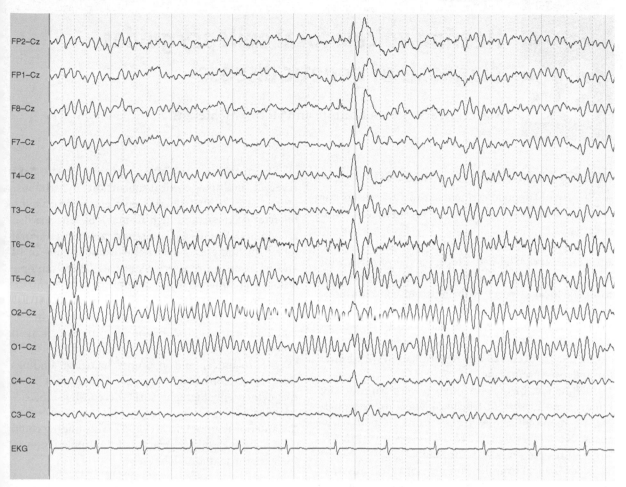

Fig. 2. EEG showing right temporal slowing and spike.

complex partial seizure was witnessed, was the diagnosis of epilepsy considered and imaging performed. It is likely that both depression and partial seizures are related to right amygdalar lesion and temporolimbic dysfunction. Often, patients experiencing strange ictal phenomena hesitate to report them due to anxiety of being diagnosed insane. On the other hand, physicians unfamiliar with complex psychic symptoms may not realize the possible epileptic nature of these symptoms.

Suggested reading

Elliott B, Joyce E, Shorvon S. Delusions, illusions and hallucinations in epilepsy: 2. Complex phenomena and psychosis. *Epilepsy Res* 2009; **85**: 172–86.

Kanner AM. Depression and epilepsy: a review of multiple facets of their close relation. *Neurol Clin* 2009; **27**: 865–80.

Kasper BS, Kerling F, Graf W, Stefan H, Pauli E. Ictal delusion of sexual transformation. *Epilepsy Behav* 2009; **16**: 356–9. Epub 2009 Aug 19.

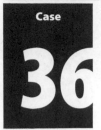

Case

36

Hearing voices: focal epilepsy guides diagnosis of genetic disease

Marcel Heers, Stefan Rampp, and Hermann Stefan

History and clinical examination

A 20-year-old female economy student presents for presurgical evaluation of her pharmacoresistant focal epilepsy.

The patient suffered from her first seizures at the age of 11 years. She had simple partial seizures with hearing of voices for several seconds, followed by complex focal seizures with impaired consciousness, making grimaces, crying, and vocalization. These episodes lasted for 1–2 minutes and occured 4–8 times per month. Just one secondarily generalized tonic–clonic seizure occurred during medication withdrawal for epilepsy monitoring.

Pregnancy, birth, and infancy were without any remarks, no history of febrile convulsions, encephalitis, or meningitis. She suffers from sleep disturbances. No factors that provoke seizures were known. No seizures are known in the family.

Neurological examination did not reveal any specific neurological deficits. She had no abnormalities of the skin, nails, or iris.

Diagnostics

During video–EEG monitoring, complex focal seizures could be recorded, which occurred during sleep. Initially, the patient had tachycardia, speaking of single words but no automatisms occurred. In two seizures, the patient subsequently had cloni of the left face, versive head movement to the left and asymmetric tonic limb posturing (figure of 4 sign) on the left side (Kotagel *et al.*, 2000). Electrophysiological seizure patterns were found initially to be bilateral with subsequent evolution of leading activity of the right frontotemporal region after 10–20 seconds.

Structural high-resolution epilepsy FLAIR MRI revealed multiple cortical/subcortical hyperintense lesions, e.g., in the superior postcentral gyrus right, bilateral occipital, and high frontal lobe left. She had an additional subtle hyperintensity anterior temporal lobe right. Some lesions were also distinguishable in T2 and in inversion recovery sequences. These multiple lesions were interpreted as multiple cortical harmatomas, which are typically caused by tuberous sclerosis.

Neuropsychological assessment showed right lateral temporal lobe dysfunction in terms of deficits in object recognition.

Electroclinical and neuropsychological findings were in concordance with spike localizations from magnetoencephalography (MEG) recordings: interictal epileptic activity recorded by MEG was localized to the anterior temporal lobe (Fig. 1). This finding could determine the epileptogenicity of the subtle lesion in the anterior temporal lobe right.

Surgery and genetic analysis

A right anterior temporal lobe resection including the amygdala was performed. one year postsurgical outcome of the patient was Engel 1A. Postoperatively the patient did not suffer from any new focal neurological deficits, although deficits in object recognition remained unchanged.

Histological analysis of the resected specimen gave hints for tuberous sclerosis. Subsequent genetic testing uncovered a mutation in TSC 1 gene in this patient.

General remarks

TSC 1 gene mutation leads to mild forms of tuberous sclerosis. These patients might not have typical stig-

---

Case Studies in Epilepsy, ed. Hermann Stefan, Elinor Ben-Menachem, Patrick Chauvel and Renzo Guerrini. Published by Cambridge University Press. © Hermann Stefan, Elinor Ben-Menachem, Patrick Chauvel and Renzo Guerrini 2012.

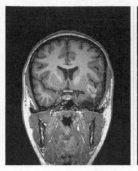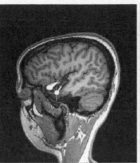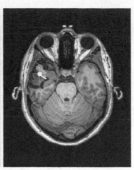

Fig. 1. Dipole localizations from epileptic spikes (white poles) coregistered with postsurgical structural MRI of the patient (dipoles are projected on the shown slice when not located in the slice). Note dipole localization within the resection volume of the patient with postsurgical outcome Engel 1A.

mata such as adenoma sebaceum, subungual skin changes, or mental retardation. These changes occur more often in patients with TSC 2 gene mutations (Napolioni *et al.*, 2009).

Special remarks

MEG can be used to determine epileptogenicity of MR positive lesions. This is of considerable help in patients with multiple, possibly epileptogenic, lesions (Stefan *et al.*, 2004; Jansen *et al.*, 2006).

Suggested reading

Jansen FE, Huiskamp G, van Huffelen AC, Identification of the epileptogenic tuber in patients with tuberous sclerosis: a comparison of high-resolution EEG and MEG. *Epilepsia* 2006; **47**: 108–14.

Kotagal P, Bleasel A, Geller E, *et al.* Lateralizing value of asymmetric tonic limb posturing observed in secondarily generalized tonic-clonic seizures. *Epilepsia* 2000; **41**: 457–62.

Napolioni V, Moavero R, Curatolo P. Recent advances in neurobiology of Tuberous Sclerosis Complex. *Brain Dev* 2009; **31**: 104–13.

Stefan H, Scheler G, Hummel C, *et al.* Magnetoencephalography (MEG) predicts focal epileptogenicity in cavernomas. *J Neurol Neurosurg Psychiatry* 2004; **75**: 1309–13.

37

Life-threatening status epilepticus due to focal cortical dysplasia

Carmen Barba and Renzo Guerrini

Clinical history

A 5-year-old girl was referred to our department for treatment of refractory lateralized status epilepticus (RSE).

General history

The child, who had a normal psychomotor development, had experienced focal motor seizures since age 2½ years. EEG showed left centro-parietal spikes, enhanced during sleep. 1.5 T brain MRI was normal. Neuropsychology revealed a normal cognitive level. A diagnosis of benign epilepsy with centro-temporal spikes (BECTS) was made.

Examination

On admission, the child was treated with intravenous midazolam and valproate. She was sedated, but was able to execute simple orders and to speak. Right-sided focal motor seizures, involving the face and then spreading to the arm and leg, appeared in series of 7–8 attacks per hour.

Special studies

Prolonged video–EEG monitoring captured seizures characterized by right hemifacial tonic contraction, followed by clonic jerking of the right arm with inconstant involvement of the homolateral leg. The ictal discharge started at the left fronto-temporo-central leads to subsequently involve the contralateral hemisphere. Repeat 1.5 T brain MRI revealed an abnormal gyral pattern, with increased cortical thickness and blurring of the gray–white matter junction, extending from the pole to the central gyrus of the left frontal lobe. Subsequent 3T brain MRI performed 2 weeks after onset of status confirmed the area of structural abnormality and also detected a clear-cut left opercular area of increased signal intensity on T2 and FLAIR-T2-weighted images.

Follow-up

Despite aggressive treatment with a combination of intravenous midazolam, phenobarbital, and phenytoin, seizure frequency and severity increased. The child was then admitted to intensive care. She was intubated and sequentially treated with intravenous ketamine and propofol, without success. Subsequent treatment with thiopentone induced a suppression-burst EEG pattern with cessation of seizures, but seizures promptly recurred upon drug tapering. Neurological examination revealed right hemiparesis. An intervening sepsis caused a significant worsening of the child's general conditions. At this moment in time, 3 weeks after the onset of status epilepticus, we decided to perform surgery urgently. Although MRI had detected an extensive malformation involving most of the left frontal lobe, from the pole to the central fissure, electroclinical findings indicated the left rolandic area as the seizure onset zone. Based on this observation, we decided to perform stereo-electroencephalography (SEEG) to precisely define the limits of the resection. We implanted 13 depth electrodes exploring the left frontal lobe and verified the exact position of each electrode on post-implantation MRI. SEEG lasted for 18 hours and assessed that the seizure onset zone involved the face and hand motor areas. We planned a tailored resection based on SEEG and MRI findings. Histology revealed focal cortical dysplasia (FCD) type IIb.

Status epilepticus stopped right after surgery. Upon awakening after surgery, the child exhibited right hemiplegia and mild language impairment. Two weeks after surgery, she was transferred to a

Case Studies in Epilepsy, ed. Hermann Stefan, Elinor Ben-Menachem, Patrick Chauvel and Renzo Guerrini. Published by Cambridge University Press. © Hermann Stefan, Elinor Ben-Menachem, Patrick Chauvel and Renzo Guerrini 2012.

rehabilitation center. Eleven months after surgery the child was seizure free on phenytoin and phenobarbital, had left hemiparesis, but was able to walk unsupported and to speak with mild fluency difficulties. Neuropsychology examination revealed attention, memory, and behavioral difficulties. EEG disclosed diffuse spike and wave discharges while awake and left temporo-parietal spikes during sleep.

Diagnosis

RSE in a child with epileptogenic FCD type IIb.

MRI and EEG findings

(a) Preoperative MRI (FLAIR). Abnormal gyral pattern, cortical thickness, and blurring of the gray–white matter junction in the left frontal lobe (white arrows) and increased signal intensity in the left frontal operculum (red arrow). (b) Postoperative MRI (T1 weighted image). Abnormal gyral pattern, cortical thickness and blurring of the gray–white matter junction in the left frontal pole (white arrow) and postsurgical vacuum area (red arrow). (c) Histopathology. Hematoxylin and eosin staining of the paraffin-embedded surgical specimen clearly demonstrates the neuropathological hallmarks of FCD IIb, i.e., dysmorphic neurons (black arrowhead) and balloon cells (black arrow). (d) SEEG recordings showing interictal spikes and waves at the contacts exploring the left opercular area. At seizure onset (red arrow), the interictal abnormalities stop and low voltage fast activity occurs at the same contacts. Electromyographic recordings disclose a contraction of the right arm starting 5 seconds after the first EEG modification (red arrowhead) (Fig. 1).

General remarks

Literature on surgery in RSE includes small case series and single case reports. Most patients exhibited focal epilepsy in relation to malformations of cortical development and underwent lesionectomies or lobar resections, usually after invasive EEG recordings. The decision to plan surgery in these patients had weighed the pros related to risks of avoiding medical complications of prolonged intensive care and the significant impairment of essential functions such as swallowing and respiration.

Surgery is an effective treatment option in a subset of patients with RSE, provided that electroclinical findings and neuroimaging provide converging evidence for a single epileptogenic zone and presurgical work-up is performed in epilepsy surgery centers with appropriate expertise.

Special remarks

In this patient, SEEG helped to precisely define the epileptogenic zone and perform a tailored resection, thus increasing the chances to obtain seizure freedom while minimising postsurgical deficits. Most reported patients were explored with intraoperative electrocorticography or prolonged invasive monitoring or were operated with extended surgical resections, without any invasive recording if hemispheric or multilobar abnormalities were present.

Our patient exhibited postsurgery hemiparesis, as expected after surgery on the sensorimotor cortex. In our patient motor and cognitive deficits rapidly improved, likely due to the tailored surgical approach sparing the leg motor as well as the language areas. The child's young age at surgery may have increased the chances of functional reorganization and favored the recovery of function. Earlier age at surgery has consistently been related to better recovery of motor and sensory function after hemispheric resections. The rate of immediate postoperative sensorimotor deficits after rolandic resections is around 60% in pediatric surgical series. However, a number of children display persistent deficits.

Determining the optimal timing for surgery in patients with RSE is a hard task as the overall clinical conditions of a given patient may be variable. Some authors have suggested a 2-week period of failed medical treatment as a sufficient delay for surgery. In our patient we planned surgery based on the failure of aggressive antiepileptic drug treatment, the occurrence of severe infections, and the progressive worsening of motor and respiratory functions. Performing SEEG required some extra time, but helped in limiting the area of resection.

Future perspectives

Follow-up studies indicate an 80% rate of seizure freedom 4 months to 5 years after epilepsy surgery for RSE. This figure might, however, represent an overestimate of the actual efficacy of surgical treatment in RSE, as failures are less likely to be reported. Future multicentric studies are needed to reach a significant number of observations, assess the overall efficacy of surgical treatment in RSE, and define the criteria for referral.

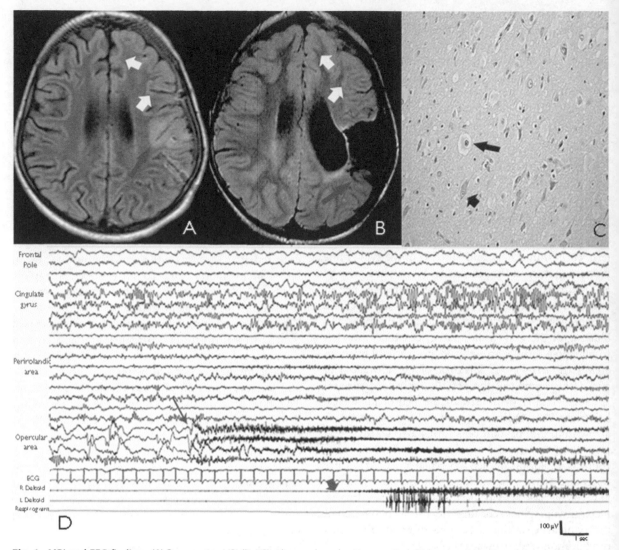

Fig. 1. MRI and EEG findings (**A**) Preoperative MRI (FLAIR). Abnormal gyral pattern, cortical thickness and blurring of the gray-white matter junction in the left frontal lobe (white arrows) and increased signal intensity in the left frontal operculum (red arrow). (**B**) Postoperative MRI (T1 weighted image). Abnormal gyral pattern, cortical thickness and blurring of the gray–white matter junction in the left frontal pole (white arrow) and postsurgical vacuum area (red arrow). (**C**) Histopathology. Hematoxylin and eosin staining of the paraffin-embedded surgical specimen clearly demonstrates the neuropathological hallmarks of FCD IIb, i.e. dysmorphic neurons (black arrowhead) and balloon cells (black arrow). (**D**) SEEG recordings showing interictal spikes and waves at the contacts exploring the left opercular area. At seizure onset (red arrow), the interictal abnormalities stop and low voltage fast activity occurs at the same contacts. Electromyographic recordings disclose a contraction of the right arm starting five seconds after the first EEG modification (red arrowhead). See color plate section.

Suggested reading

Alexopoulos A, Lachhwani DK, Gupta A, *et al.* Resective surgery to treat refractory status epilepticus in children with focal epileptogenesis. *Neurology* 2005; **64**: 567–70.

Benifla M, Sala F Jr, Jane J, *et al.* Neurosurgical management of intractable rolandic epilepsy in children: role of resection in eloquent cortex. *J Neurosurg Pediatr* 2009; **4**: 199–216.

Choi JT, Vining EPG, Mori S, Bastian AM. Sensorimotor function and sensorimotor tracts after hemispherectomy. *Neuropsychologia* 2010; **48**: 1192–9.

Cross JH, Jayakar P, Nordii D, *et al.* Proposed criteria for referral and evaluation of children for epilepsy surgery: recommendations of the subcommission for pediatric epilepsy surgery. *Epilepsia* 2006; **47**: 952–9.

Desbiens R, Berkovic SF, Dubeau F, Andermann F, Laxer KD, Harvey S. Life-threatening focal status epilepticus due to occult cortical dysplasia. *Arch. Neurol* 1993; **50**: 695–700.

D'Giano C, Garcia MD, Pomata H, Rabinowicz AL. Treatment of refractory partial status epilepticus with multiple subpial transection: a case report. *Seizure* 2001; **10**: 382–5.

Duane DC, Ng YT, Rekate HL, *et al.* Treatment of refractory status epilepticus with hemispherectomy. *Epilepsia* 2004; **45**: 1001–4.

Gorman DJ, Shields WD, Shewmon DA, *et al.* Neurosurgical treatment of refractory status epilepticus. *Epilepsia* 1992; **33**: 546–9.

Krsek P, Tichy M, Belsan T, *et al.* Life-saving epilepsy surgery for status epilepticus caused by cortical dysplasia. *Epileptic Disord* 2002; **4**: 203–8.

Lhatoo SD, Alexopoulos A. The surgical treatment of status epilepticus. *Epilepsia* 2007; **48**: 61–5.

Ma X, Liporace J, O'Connor MJ, Sperling MR. Neurosurgical treatment of medically intractable status epilepticus. *Epilepsy Res* 2001; **46**: 33–8.

Ng YT, Kim HL, Wheless JW. Successful neurosurgical treatment of childhood complex partial status epilepticus with focal resection. *Epilepsia* 2003; **44**: 468–71.

Rossetti AO, Logroscino G, Bromfield EB. Refractory status epilepticus: effect of treatment aggressiveness on prognosis. *Arch Neurol* 2005; **62**: 1698–702.

Vendrame M, Loddenkemper T. Surgical treatment of refractory status epilepticus in children: candidate selection and outcome. *Semin Pediatr Neurol* 2010; **17**: 182–9.

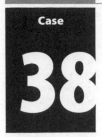

Childhood occipital idiopathic epilepsy

Carmen Barba and Renzo Guerrini

Clinical history

A 4-year-old boy was admitted to our unit 2 hours after his first seizure, which was characterized by vomiting, headache, and unresponsiveness. The attack occurred during sleep and lasted 25 minutes.

General history

Family history for febrile seizures. Normal psycho-motor development.

Examination

Neurological examination was normal.

Special studies

The child underwent repeated video–EEG recordings, while awake and asleep (10–20 International Electrode Placement System, including the Oz electrode) with intermittent photic stimulation (IPS) and hyperventilation. EEG showed normal background activity with bilateral temporo-occipital spikes and wave discharges, with right predominance and activated during sleep. IPS evoked no EEG change. 1.5 T brain MRI was normal.

During a routine follow-up EEG, the child happened to manifest his third seizure, which occurred during sleep (stage 2, non-REM sleep). At seizure onset, interictal EEG abnormalities ceased to be replaced after 2 minutes by an irregular rhythmic 4 Hz activity building up over the right occipital leads and rapidly involving the contralateral occipital region. Six minutes after its onset, the ictal discharge became more diffuse and with sharper outline, especially on right occipital and Oz leads. Seven minutes and 30 seconds after onset, the respirogram started to show recurrent apneas lasting 6–7 seconds each.

After 10 minutes 20 seconds, the child opened his eyes, blinking for few seconds and started to chew and retch, and turned his head and eyes to the left. The behavioral arousal was accompanied in the EEG by a spike discharge that gradually spread to both hemispheres, with intermingled faster rhythms on the right occipital leads and at Oz. At 11 minutes 40 seconds, the child started vomiting and deviated his eyes and head to the left. He was able to name objects, describe their colors, and perform simple motor tasks upon request. He repetitively tried to turn his head towards his father on the right side, but, after a few seconds, again deviated his head and eyes to the left. Vomiting reappeared intermittently four times over the following 10 minutes. At 22 minutes, the child was unable to sit and pick up his arms, but continued to correctly answer simple questions. The seizure was stopped 34 minutes after its onset using endorectal diazepam.

Follow-up

After his first seizure, the child was discharged without treatment. He experienced five more seizures mainly during sleep, characterized by eye and head deviation to the left, retching, intermittent vomiting, and progressive unresponsiveness. After his second seizure, carbamazepine was started. Due to inefficacy in controlling seizures and increase of interictal EEG discharges, carbamazepine was switched to valproate. The last seizure occurred at age 5 years. At the last follow-up, at age 7, no EEG abnormalities were recorded.

EEG findings (Fig. 1)

(a) At seizure onset, during sleep, interictal temporo-parieto-occipital spikes cease (red arrow). (b) At 1 minute and 30 seconds, bilateral occipital 4 Hz rhythmic activity is recognizable (red arrow). (c) At 7 minutes, the

Case Studies in Epilepsy, ed. Hermann Stefan, Elinor Ben-Menachem, Patrick Chauvel and Renzo Guerrini. Published by Cambridge University Press. © Hermann Stefan, Elinor Ben-Menachem, Patrick Chauvel and Renzo Guerrini 2012.

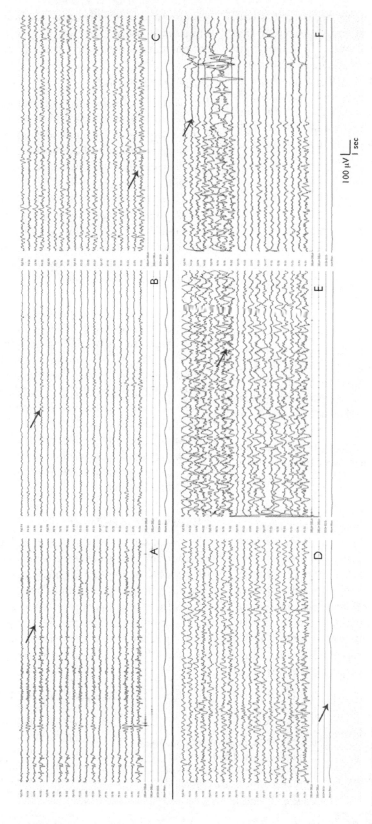

100 µV | 1 sec

Fig. 1. EEG findings

(a) At seizure onset, during sleep, interictal temporo-parieto-occipital spikes cease (arrow). (b) At 1 minute and 30 seconds, bilateral occipital 4 Hz rhythmic activity is recognisable (arrow). (c) At 7 minutes, the ictal discharge has become more diffuse and sharp, especially on the right occipital and Oz electrode (arrow). (d) At 9 minutes 30 seconds, the respirogram documents an apnea lasting 6 seconds (arrow). (e) At 24 minutes, EEG shows a diffuse spike discharge, with intermingled faster rhythms on the right occipital leads (arrow) and at the Oz electrode (Electrocardiogram (EKG) and respirogram are poorly connected). (f) At 32 minutes, after diazepam administration (arrow), EEG shows diffuse flattening (EKG and respirogram are poorly connected).

ictal discharge has become more diffuse and sharp, especially on the right occipital and Oz electrode (red arrow). (d) At 9 minutes 30 seconds, the respirogram documents an apnea lasting 6 seconds (red arrow). (e) At 24 minutes, EEG shows a diffuse spike discharge, with intermingled faster rhythms on the right occipital leads (red arrow) and at the Oz electrode (Electrocardiogram (EKG) and respirogram are poorly connected). (f) At 32 minutes, after diazepam administration (red arrow), EEG shows diffuse flattening (EKG and respirogram are poorly connected) (Fig. 1).

Diagnosis

Early onset childhood occipital idiopathic epilepsy.

General remarks

Childhood occipital idiopathic epilepsy was originally described by Gastaut in 1982 as an idiopathic partial epilepsy with visual seizures (illusions, elementary hallucinations, ictal blindness) evolving either to hemiclonic or complex partial seizures, with or without secondary generalization, with an age of onset between 15 months and 17 years. In around 25% of Gastaut's patients, a migraine-type postictal headache was reported. Interictal EEG showed normal background activity, with high amplitude, unilateral or bilateral, synchronous or asynchronous, occipital spike-and-wave discharges, facilitated by eye closure. Outcome was generally favorable with remission before adulthood.

A subset of children with ICOE present brief or prolonged sleep-related seizures characterized by tonic eye and head deviation, vomiting and eventually hemiclonic spread or secondary generalization. The age at seizure onset is between 2 and 8 years. Prognosis is excellent with remission by the age of 12 and with most children having suffered only one seizure. This form of early onset idiopathic occipital epilepsy is also referred to as "Panayiotopoulos syndrome" or benign childhood seizure susceptibility syndrome. Due to its favorable outcome and the rarity of seizures, chronic antiepileptic medication is not recommended unless seizures become frequent or are accompanied by secondary generalization.

Special remarks

In this case ictal video–EEG recordings helped define the electroclinical pattern and make a diagnosis. Due to the rarity of seizures and the good prognosis, only a few single case studies have documented ictal recordings in children with childhood occipital idiopathic epilepsy.

The clinical history and the electroclinical pattern in our patient strongly suggested a diagnosis of early onset childhood occipital idiopathic epilepsy: seizures started at age 4, occurred rarely and were prolonged (more than 30 minutes), usually occurring during sleep or upon falling asleep. Clinical features included eye and head deviation contralaterally to the ictal discharge, intermittent vomiting, and progressive unresponsiveness. The ictal discharge originated from the posterior temporal-parieto-occipital regions, with a clear occipital predominance and preceded the first clinical manifestation by several minutes.

An interesting additional clinical feature in this syndrome is the waxing and waning of clinical manifestations during a seizure such as eye and head deviation and unresponsiveness, which might also lead experienced staff to underestimate the real duration of the seizures, unless simultaneous EEG recording is available.

Future perspectives

The initial seizure of early onset childhood occipital epilepsy can be misdiagnosed as onset of an encephalitic process, as migraine, syncope, or gastroenteritis. The definition of electroclinical features in large series of children with this type of epilepsy might help to define more specific criteria for early diagnosis, avoiding unnecessary complementary investigations and potentially harmful treatments.

Suggested reading

Demirbilek V, Dervent V. Panayiotopoulos syndrome: video–EEG illustration of a typical seizure. *Epileptic Disord* 2004; **6**: 121–4.

Ferrie CD, Beaumanoir A, Guerrini R, *et al.* Early-onset benign occipital seizure susceptibility syndrome. *Epilepsia* 1997; **38**: 285–93.

Gastaut H. A new type of epilepsy: benign partial epilepsy of childhood with occipital spike-waves. *Clin Electroenceph* 1982; **13**: 13–22.

Gastaut H, Roger J, Bureau M. Benign epilepsy of childhood with occipital paroxysms. Up-date. In J Roger, M Bureau, C Dravet, *et al.*, eds. *Epileptic Syndromes in Infancy, Childhood and Adolescence.* 2nd edn. London: John Libbey, 1992; 201–17.

Guerrini R, Belmonte A, Veggiotti P, Mattia D, Bonanni P. Delayed appearance of interictal EEG abnormalities in early onset childhood epilepsy with occipital paroxysms. *Brain Dev* 1997; **19**: 343–6.

Panayiotopoulos CP. Benign nocturnal childhood occipital epilepsy: a new syndrome with nocturnal seizures, tonic deviation of the eyes, and vomiting. *J Child Neurol* 1989; **4**: 43–8.

Panayiotopoulos CP, Michael M, Sanders S, Valeta T, Koutroumanidis M. Benign childhood focal epilepsies: assessment of established and newly recognized syndromes. *Brain* 2008; **131**: 2264–86.

Salanova V, Andermann F, Olivier A, Rasmussen T, Quesney LF. Occipital lobe epilepsy: electroclinical manifestations, electrocorticography, cortical stimulation and outcome in 42 patients treated between 1930 and 1991. Surgery of occipital lobe epilepsy. *Brain* 1992; **115**: 1655–80.

Specchio N, Trivisano M, Claps D, et al. Documentation of autonomic seizure and autonomic status epilepticus with ictal EEG in Panayiotopoulos syndrome. *Epilepsy Behav* 2010; **19**: 383–93.

Thomas P, Arzimanoglou A, Aicardi J. Benign idiopathic occipital epilepsy: report of a case of the early benign type. *Epileptic Disord* 2003; **5**: 57–9.

Vigevano F, Lispi ML, Ricci S. Early onset benign occipital susceptibility syndrome: video–EEG documentation of an illustrative case. *Clin Neurophysiol* 2000; **111**: 81–6.

Williamson PD, Thadani VM, Darcey TM, et al. Occipital lobe epilepsy: clinical characteristics, seizure spread patterns, and results of surgery. *Ann Neurol* 1992; **31**: 3–13.

39

Unconscious: never again work above a meter?

Tobias Knieß

Clinical history

6.46 am.: A bus driver finds the unconscious Mr. L.A lying on the ground at a bus stop.

6.52 am: Emergency services arrive. L.A. has regained consciousness, but his reaction is slowed.

7.10 am: During transport to hospital, he again loses consciousness for several minutes, accompanied by bilateral convulsions in arms and legs. The emergency physician injects 10 mg diazepam.

Personal history

L.A. is working as an apprentice painter. His parents are separated, he is in a relationship, and claims to have a lot of stress at work. He does not take drugs, and is a casual drinker. His medical history is unremarkable, there had been no complications at his birth, no traumatic brain injuries, no epilepsy in the family history, no provocative factors.

First examination results

On arrival at the local hospital's emergency department, he is first examined. It is confirmed that his reactions are slowed (GCS 12), and he is suffering from amnesia with no memory of what had happened. Temperature, blood pressure, glucose, and oxygen levels are normal. No neurologicalal focal deficits (NIHSS 0), no injuries.

Later examinations

Laboratory checks including drug screening: normal results.

Emergency CCT: no bleeding, no ischemia, no tumors, no fractures.

Early EEG (8.00 am): no lesions, no epileptic activity.

Sleep derivation EEG the following day: no lesions, no epileptic activity.

Long-term ECG: sine rhythm.

Daily blood glucose profile: unremarkable.

Schellong test: no signs for orthostatic dysregulation.

3 T MRI with contrast agents and thin-layer: no morphological brain lesions, no dysplasia, no Ammonshorn sclerosis, no cavernome, no migration deficits (Fig. 1).

Later history

One night before release from hospital, the incident is repeated, convulsions in arms and legs, open and closed eyes, random actions. Convulsions can be interrupted by addressing patient, L.A. replies adequately. He reports his partner is pregnant, third month, he is afraid to inform his parents, and fears for the future. Psychosomatic consultation follows.

Diagnosis

Non-epileptic psychogenic seizures under acute reactive stress disorder.

General remarks

Without initial second-party anamnesis and probable second seizure, suspected manifestation of epilepsy with complex focal tonic–clonic seizure. Intensive additional aperitif diagnostics could not sufficiently support the diagnosis of epilepsy. Anticonvulsive therapy was not appropriate. On the night before planned release from hospital with suspected diagnosis of convulsive syncope another incident was observed by trained personnel. Confirmed as prolonged non-epileptic psychogenic seizure. During search for psycho-dynamic triggers, L.A. hesitantly

Case Studies in Epilepsy, ed. Hermann Stefan, Elinor Ben-Menachem, Patrick Chauvel and Renzo Guerrini. Published by Cambridge University Press. © Hermann Stefan, Elinor Ben-Menachem, Patrick Chauvel and Renzo Guerrini 2012.

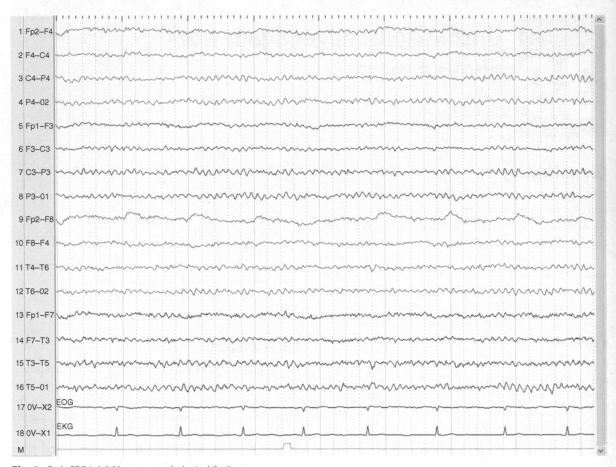

Fig. 1. Early-EEG L.A.8:00 am: no pathological findings.

reported the unwanted pregnancy of his girlfriend, he was afraid of the future and afraid of explaining the situation to his parents. Consulted psychosomatic doctors made diagnosis of acute reactive adjustment disorder with dissociative non-epileptic psychogenic seizures. Psychotherapy with conflict resolution in- or outpatient was recommended. L.A. was released without anticonvulsives after many supportive discussions, including his mother and father.

Further remarks

Early psychotherapy as well as solution of the conflict and short progression of disorder support positive prognosis.

Occupational health concerns: as painter, L.A. works on ladders and scaffoldings; seizures (even non-epileptic) with disrupted reaction and consciousness fulfill danger category "C" according to German employer's liability insurance association, prohibiting unsecured work above the height of 1 meter (3 feet). Additionally, L.A. is not capable of driving until further notice. There is significant danger that he will not be able to continue his apprenticeship.

Future perspectives

L.A. has been advised to contact an epilepsy advice specialist and/or the integration service for advice regarding measures securing his apprenticeship or providing alternative occupation.

40

A patient's patience

Hermann Stefan

Clinical history

A 47-year-old female patient sustained a head trauma with epidural hematoma, which was operated. During the rehabilitation phase, focal clonic seizures in the left side of the face as well as fluctuating slowing of reaction and disorientation occurred. The dyscognitive seizures secondarily generalized to bilateral convulsive seizures.

Treatment

Treatment with carbamazepine could not control the seizure and was associated with marked tiredness. Seizures persisted occurring every second or third day, lasting from 30 seconds to hours. Therefore, the anticonvulsive medication had been changed from carbamazepine to levetiracetam monotherapy. Under this therapy, seizure frequency markedly reduced, but seizures still occurred lasting up to 2 hours. Seizures developed during the night emerging with motoric signs (convulsions of both arms and left leg), tachycardia as well as panic. These seizures repeatedly occurred enduring up to 2 hours. In addition to the seizures, the patient had difficulties in concentration, memory function, and was exhausted. Because of this difficulty in treating the epilepsy, the patient was investigated anew.

Neurological examination

Visual field left sided reduced, Romberg test positive with tendency to fall backwards and to the right side, left-sided dysdiadochokinesis and hypesthesia left face side and left hand.

EEG showed irregular alpha background activity with intermittent theta parieto-temporal right. No epileptiform activity.

Due to the neurological and psychiatric deficits, the patient had a reduced working time of 13 hours per week.

Diagnosis

Follow-up

Because of the uncontrolled seizure activity in addition to levetiracetam, lacosamide was introduced. The dose of levetiracetam was 1250-0-1500 mg and lacosamide was added with a dose of 50 mg in the morning every 2 weeks up to a target dose of 250 mg per day. Especially in the first week, but also during each increase of dosage, dizziness, headache and disturbance of coordination reappeared. These symptoms disappeared after several days and occurred again after an increase of 50 mg lacosamide several times. These side effects made it difficult for the patient to continue with this drug. When the patient recognized that the side effects decreased after some days, she decided to continue the drug intake despite transient side effects. Two months after onset of lacosamide treatment, dizziness had completely disappeared, and tiredness had also improved. Two months after onset of lacosamide treatment additive to levetiracetam, seizure frequency had reduced by about 60%. Following this, her working capacity and efficiency increased considerably.

General comment

The motivation, the patience, endurance, and adherence, of the patient were important preconditions for treatment success. It is important to note that central nervous side effects may be transitory.

Case Studies in Epilepsy, ed. Hermann Stefan, Elinor Ben-Menachem, Patrick Chauvel and Renzo Guerrini. Published by Cambridge University Press. © Hermann Stefan, Elinor Ben-Menachem, Patrick Chauvel and Renzo Guerrini 2012.

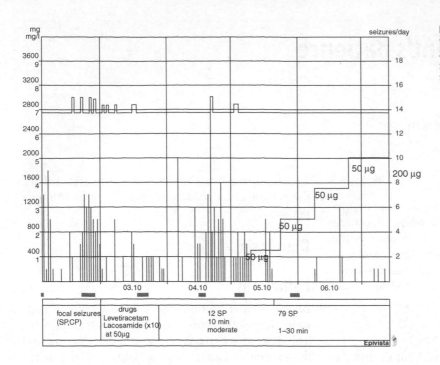

Fig. 1. Long-term follow-up during treatment with levetiracetam, lacosamide. Adding lacosamide to levetiracetam in small doses led to marked reduction of seizure frequency and duration.

The case shows that it can be worthwhile continuing with a treatment and not to switch too soon to another anticonvulsive drug. After recognizing that the side effects are transitory, a further increase of lacosamide up to 175–0–150 mg/day could be applied and the dose rate of levetiracetam reduced to 1250–0–1250 mg in order to reduce the total drug load (Fig. 1).

This combination treatment led to a further improvement with shortened seizures and improving performance in everyday life.

Special remark

Whereas in former times the advantages of monotherapies dominated, an early use of newer anticonvulsants without relevant interaction potential or cognitive side is possible. Concerning the selection of anticonvulsive drugs for combination therapy, the mechanism of action is also discussed. In this case the combination of a sodium blocker (lacosamide) and a non-sodium channel blocker (levetiracetam) was successful. It is currently being discussed whether this could be a principle for rational polytherapy.

Suggested reading

Deckers CL, Hekster YA, Keyser A, et al. Monotherapy versus polytherapy for epilepsy: a multicenter double-blind randomized study. *Epilepsia* 2001; **42**: 1387–94.

Sake LK, Hebert D, Isojärvi J, et al. A pooled analysis of lacosamide clinical trial data grouped by mechanism of action of concomitant antiepileptic drugs. *CNS Drugs* 2010; **24**: 1055–68.

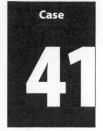

Case

41

Idiopathic absence epilepsy: unusual AED consumption successful

Elinor Ben-Menachem

This man was born in 1957. His father was diagnosed with absence epilepsy as a child, but was seizure free as an adult. As far as we know, the absences started in 1963 when he was 6 years old, but he was finally diagnosed at the age of 12 with absence epilepsy after he had had his first generalized tonic–clonic (?) (GTC) seizures. An EEG at that time showed short 3 second spike and wave activity during hyperventilation only. In 1979 he complained of myoclonic jerks on awakening and drop attacks in 1981. By 1984 he was having one to two GTCs a week and many absences a day. He had been tried on many different AED combinations until that point: carbamazepine, phenytoin, ethosuximide, primidone, phenobarbital, valproate, diamox, and clonazepam, and was never seizure free. In other words, he had tried all the AEDs available at that time alone and in combination.

In 1984 he was admitted to our hospital to try to convert him over to a high dose of valproate monotherapy, as information was available that valproate would be the drug of choice for absence epilepsy with GTC (Bruni et al., 1980). At the time of admission he was receiving ethosuximide as well as phenytoin. In the hospital he was converted to valproate 2100 mg/day and phenytoin was down titrated. He did not improve with valproate and phenytoin had to be reinstated because of the increase in GTCs. Because of his seizure situation and lack of effect of valproate, he finally left the hospital on phenytoin and ethosuximide. He then had about two to three GTCs per month and a few absences per day in 1985. In that situation he could actually work and get married and start to raise a family.

In 1985 he participated in a gabapentin vs. placebo trial for primary generalized seizures and he did not improve (Chadwick et al., 1996). He continued on gabapentin anyway and then participated in a similar study with lamotrigine, also with no reduction in seizure frequency. According to our current knowledge based mostly on anecdotal reports, lamotrigine should have caused some improvement in his situation (Posner et al., 2005). This was, however, not the case here even though his EEG continued to show the same pattern and a CT scan was normal.

He was then implanted with a vagus nerve stimulator (VNS) in 1992 and this did result in fewer GTCs and fewer absences. Before VNS, he had 26 GTCs/year and 23 726 absences/year. One year after VNS implantation he had 18 GTCs/year and 32 absences! Although he was very happy with the result, the patient was still not seizure free. He was dependent on his family, the goodwill at work and, of course, he could not drive a car. Therefore, he participated in another clinical trial, this time with topiramate. At that time, he was taking phenytoin, gabapentin, and clobazam as well as VNS. He was started on topiramate and became seizure free on a dose of 125 mg/day, although we know today that topiramate is not especially effective on absences (Ormrod and McClellan, 2001). VNS was stopped in 1999 without any negative consequences. Gabapentin and clobazam were stopped successfully. However, attempts to reduce phenytoin did not succeed and every time phenytoin was reduced to just 25 mg, he had a new seizure.

The patient is now on phenytoin and topiramate and has been seizure free since 2002. His EEG has normalized completely and he now drives a car and lives a normal life with his family after suffering from seizures for 45 years.

Lesson to learn
General remarks

Achieving seizure freedom in refractory epilepsy patients is not an easy task. It may take years of effort

---

Case Studies in Epilepsy, ed. Hermann Stefan, Elinor Ben-Menachem, Patrick Chauvel and Renzo Guerrini. Published by Cambridge University Press. © Hermann Stefan, Elinor Ben-Menachem, Patrick Chauvel and Renzo Guerrini 2012.

from the physician as well as from the patient who should be encouraged not to give up during the process. Never stop trying is the main message and sometimes therapies that we cannot imagine would work can surprisingly make the patient seizure free.

Neurologists should try to keep their refractory patients and follow them closely. Today, many patients are evaluated by different doctors, making it is almost impossible to finally arrive at a useful therapy.

Suggested reading

Bruni J, Wilder BJ, Bauman AW, Willmore LJ. Clinical efficacy and long-term effects of valproic acid therapy on spike-and-wave discharges. *Neurology* 1980; **30**: 42–6.

Chadwick D, Leiderman DB, Sauermann W, Alexander J,

Garofalo E. Gabapentin in generalized seizures. *Epilepsy Res* 1996; **25**: 191–7.

Ormrod D, McClellan K. Topiramate: a review of its use in childhood epilepsy. *Paediatr Drugs* 2001; **3**: 293–319.

Posner EB, Mohamed K, Marson AG. Ethosuximide, sodium valproate or lamotrigine for absence seizures in children and adolescents. *Cochrane Database Syst Rev.* 2003; (**3**): CD003032. Review. Update in: Cochrane Database Syst Rev 2005; (**4**): CD003032.

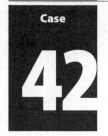

Woman with gastric reflux – careful with combinations of medications

Elinor Ben-Menachem

This is a woman born in 1946 by normal delivery. She had epilepsy since she was a child and her earliest memory is from the age of four. Her epilepsy was refractory to medication at that time and she was diagnosed with refractory focal seizures, which often generalized to tonic–clonic seizures. After epilepsy surgical evaluation, she was operated on in 1983 with a left anterior temporal lobectomy for mesial temporal lobe epilepsy.

Unfortunately, the surgery was unsuccessful and she continued to have both focal and generalized seizures, approximately one generalized seizure every other week and two focal seizures per week. She experienced auras daily and so was always afraid she would have a seizure.

During the years she had tried the following therapies: carbamazepine, vigabatrin, lamotrigine, topiramate, tiagabine, clobazam, and levetiracetam. She received a vagus nerve stimulator in 1998, but it had only a marginal effect, but she is afraid to stop the generator. At the moment, however, we are slowly reducing stimulation strength (mA).

In 2002 she started a trial of lacosamide. The study was very successful for her and the generalized seizures disappeared. In 2010 she was having only infrequent focal seizures (one every 2–3 months and one or two auras per month).

In addition to lacosamide, she is also taking carbamazepine and levetiracetam and vagus nerve stimulation.

The problem and lesson

In 2005, she complained of gastric reflux and she therefore went to her primary care physician. He gave her the newest proton pump inhibitor, which was 20 mg of Nexium (esomeprazol). This drug is metabolized by CYP2 C19 and CYP3 A4.

After 3 days she could not stand on her feet. She complained of extreme dizziness and needed to hold on to her husband when she walked. She went to the emergency room of her local hospital where a blood concentration of carbamazepine was taken. Normally, her concentration was 30 µmol/l but now it had increased to 60 µmol/l.

She was subsequently hospitalized, the esomeprazol was withdrawn, and the carbamazepine concentration returned to normal and the side effects disappeared.

General remarks

Carbamazepine is metabolized by the liver enzymes CYP 3A4, CYP2C, CYP 2D6 and transport protein p-glycoprotein and induces these enzymes (Masubuchi et al., 2001). Drugs that have the same metabolic pathway can cause a steep rise in the levels of CBZ as well as carbamazepine-10,11-epoxide.

Therefore, the physician must always check carefully not to combine two drugs that are metabolized by CYP 3A4 or CYP2C or CYP 2D6, especially if one is carbamazepine, as this will invariably cause interactions and an increase of CBZ concentration.

Special remarks

In 2009 the patient developed high blood pressure and again was given a new drug (metoprolol), this time for hypertension. The same reaction occurred, but because she remembered the incident in 2005 she was able to immediately call her doctor, stop the metoprolol and she recovered after 3 days. Metoprolol is mainly metabolized by CYP 2D6, but a minor part is metabolized by CYP 2D6, and a minor part of

Case Studies in Epilepsy, ed. Hermann Stefan, Elinor Ben-Menachem, Patrick Chauvel and Renzo Guerrini. Published by Cambridge University Press. © Hermann Stefan, Elinor Ben-Menachem, Patrick Chauvel and Renzo Guerrini 2012.

carbamazepine is metabolized by the same enzyme, which was enough to cause carbamazepine toxicity. She is currently doing well on enalapril, which does not interact with carbamazepine.

Other common interactions due to CYP 3A4 with CBZ are erythromycin, warfarin, contraceptive pills, fluoxetin, dextropropoxifen, and grapefruit juice.

Suggested reading

Masubuchi Y, Nakano T, Ose A, Horie T. Differential selectivity in carbamazepine-induced inactivation of cytochrome P450 enzymes in rat and human liver. *Arch Toxicol* 2001; **75**: 538–43.

Patsalos PN, Perucca E. Clinically important drug interactions in epilepsy: general features and interactions between antiepileptic drugs. *Lancet Neurol* 2003; **2**: 347–56.

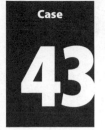

Case
43

An example of both pharmacodynamic and pharmacokinetic interactions

Elinor Ben-Menachem

History

This is a 60-year-old man with hemifacial atrophy. He was a sea captain, but developed focal onset epilepsy at the age of 43 and had to retire. He finally had epilepsy surgery with a left-sided temporal lobe resection but without improvement of his seizures, which continued as before. He even had several bouts of status epilepticus. He was medicated with carbamazepine 1600 mg/day and phenytoin 300 mg/day. Topiramate was added to his medication in 1997 and his seizures improved, so that he has not had status epilepticus since then and has fewer generalized seizures as well as focal seizures. After 3 months on a stable dose of topiramate, he began to complain of dizziness and started having hallucinations, seeing small animals on his body and people and animals in the room. He also became quite agitated.

Examination

The blood concentration of phenytoin was found to have increased to 110 μmol/l from 70 μmol/l when topiramate (300 mg/day) was added, although the dose of phenytoin was not changed. The concentration of carbamazepine did not change. When the phenytoin dose was reduced so that the concentration was again 60 μmol/l, his mental state and dizziness improved. The concentration of phenytoin is now 28 μmol/l and he remains on topiramate and carbamazepine without side effects. We have plans to stop phenytoin, as his seizure frequency has improved and does not seem to depend on phenytoin.

General remarks

This is an example of how side effects can be additive.

Special remarks

Whereas a high concentration of phenytoin does not usually cause extensive psychiatric side effects, the addition of topiramate inhibited the metabolism of phenytoin, thus causing a rise in the blood concentration. When adding new drugs, which induce or inhibit the same cytochromes (CYT2C19) as the initial antiepileptic drug (AED), the physician must be aware of potential pharmacodynamic and pharmacokinetic effects, both positive ones as in improving seizure control and negative ones as in accentuating and eliciting side effects (Patsalos and Perucca, 2003).

Six cytochrome enzymes metabolize topiramate. Both topiramate and phenytoin have common pathways so interactions would not be surprising. The lesson learned is to control the blood concentration of phenytoin when adding topiramate to the antiepileptic drug regimen. Another example of both pharmacodynamic and pharmacokinetic interaction is a combination of lamotrigine and valproate (Pisani et al., 1999).

Suggested reading

Patsalos PN, Perucca E. Clinically important drug interactions in epilepsy: general features and interactions between antiepileptic drugs. *Lancet Neurol* 2003; **2**: 347–56.

Pisani F, Oteri G, M.F. *et al.* The efficacy of valproate–lamotrigine comedication in refractory complex partial seizures: evidence for a pharmacodynamic interaction. *Epilepsia* 1999: **40**: 1141–6.

Case Studies in Epilepsy, ed. Hermann Stefan, Elinor Ben-Menachem, Patrick Chauvel and Renzo Guerrini. Published by Cambridge University Press. © Hermann Stefan, Elinor Ben-Menachem, Patrick Chauvel and Renzo Guerrini 2012.

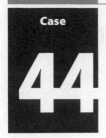

Never give up trying to find the right medication even in patients who are refractory

Elinor Ben-Menachem

History

This woman was a healthy young person until 1968, when she had a serious encephalitis at the age of 24. The only sequel after she recovered was refractory epilepsy. At the time of her encephalitis, she was married and had two young children. She was never able to work because of her epilepsy and her mother-in-law who lived close by helped her with the children and the housework. Her EEG has always shown a left temporal lobe focus and the most recent MRI showed small vessel disease (she was a chain smoker) as well as bilateral changes in the gray matter of the left anterior temporal lobe, but she was deemed not suitable for epilepsy surgery because of anticipated potential memory loss.

In an attempt to reduce her seizures, many antiepileptic drugs were tried in monotherapy and in combination. Still she persisted with four to six generalized tonic–clonic seizures monthly. The earlier AEDs tried were carbamazepine, phenytoin, phenobarbital, vigabatrin, lamotrigine, and topiramate. She was on levetiracetam monotherapy when we started to consider vagus nerve stimulation. In parallel, she was given the opportunity to participate in a lacosamide clinical trial, which she preferred to try before going on to implantation of a vagus nerve stimulator.

She started the clinical trial in 2003 and is still continuing on 400 mg of lacosamide as well as levetiracetam. The results have been remarkable, as she has been seizure free for 7 years with the exception of a generalized seizure approximately once a year when she is with her husband during the hunting season and has to help skin the deer or moose. She is trying to avoid this situation and has been successful for the last 2 years.

General remarks

Schiller and Najjar (2008) made a prospective study analyzing the probability of becoming seizure free or even being a responder after trying one to seven antiepileptic drugs previously, According to this author, this patient who had tried seven antiepileptic drugs without remarkable success would have a low probablility of ever becoming seizure free or even a responder (>50% seizure reduction). Still she did become seizure free on her eighth drug while she participated in a clinical trial, except when she has to clean a deer or moose.

Special remarks

One must remember never to give up and be complacent with regard to patients' seizure rate. There will always be the next drug available or a clinical trial along with the hope of finally achieving seizure freedom.

Suggested reading

Schiller Y, Najjar Y. Quantifying the response to antiepileptic drugs: effect of past treatment history. *Neurology* 2008; **1**: 54–65.

Case Studies in Epilepsy, ed. Hermann Stefan, Elinor Ben-Menachem, Patrick Chauvel and Renzo Guerrini. Published by Cambridge University Press. © Hermann Stefan, Elinor Ben-Menachem, Patrick Chauvel and Renzo Guerrini 2012.

Case 45

Juvenile myoclonic epilepsy and seizure aggravation

Elinor Ben-Menachem

This man was born in 1981 and had his first generalized tonic–clonic seizure at the age of 13, followed by myoclonic jerks especially in the mornings. He came to Sweden from Iraq as an adult in 2005. While in Iraq, he was started on phenobarbital and carbamazepine in 1994. His seizures continued with one or two generalized tonic–clonic seizures per month and myoclonic jerks daily especially in the morning. Sometimes he would fall during the myoclonias. This was the situation when he came to Sweden.

His EEG showed bilateral synchronized paroxysmal activity typical for generalized epilepsy. His CT and MRI studies were normal.

During his time in Sweden, he was continually unemployed, but married a woman from Iraq whom he took to Sweden. She rapidly learned Swedish and has been able to help him and has kept the seizure diary. He has not been able to go to Swedish language classes or job training because of seizures and myoclonias.

The first physician he met in Sweden switched his drugs to a combination of lamotrigine and valproate. The generalized tonic–clonic seizures disappeared, but the myoclonias continued, worse than ever. Because lamotrigine is known to cause an aggravation of myoclonias (Panayiotopoulos, 2001), the drug was stopped in 2007, and he just continued on valproate monotherapy with fewer myoclonias, but after a few months some generalized seizures reappeared.

Levetiracetam was added to the valproate in 2008 with improvement, but he was not seizure free. He was still afraid to go out alone and attempts to go to school resulted in seizures at school. He spent most of the day in his apartment while his wife attended school.

In August 2008 in a desperate attempt to improve the situation, he was started on clobazam, which is not a licensed drug in Sweden, but is in many European countries and Canada. The treatment now consisted of valproate 600 mg/day, levetiracetam 2000 mg/day and clobazam 20 mg/day. The addition of clobazam made him seizure free from the time he took the first tablet. He has now been seizure free from both myoclonias and generalized tonic–clonic seizures for 1½ years, has started back at school and is planning to get his driver's license. His EEG has normalized completely.

General remarks

There are two lessons to be learnt in this case. First of all, lamotrigine, although a popular drug for juvenile myoclonic epilepsy, has not been tested in a clinical trial for JME. In fact, there are reports of seizure aggravation and increase of myoclonias with lamotrigine, so the physician should remember this caveat and replace lamotrigine if the patient does not become entirely seizure free (Panayiopoulos, 2001). Also, carbamazepine and phenobarbital are contraindicated for juvenile myoclonic epilepsy and should not be considered (Glauser et al., 2006). They can cause seizure exacerbation. It is therefore important for the physician to have the correct diagnosis when starting AED therapy.

Clobazam (Canadian Clobazam Cooperative Group, 1991) is a benzodiazepine derivative, which has been used as an antiepileptic drug since 1984, and was approved in Canada and several EU countries as well as Japan and India for adjunctive use in tonic–clonic, complex partial, and myoclonic seizures. This AED is often forgotten when physicians consider antiepileptic drugs, but it is an important adjunctive therapy, especially when patients do not respond to other antiepileptic drugs.

Case Studies in Epilepsy, ed. Hermann Stefan, Elinor Ben-Menachem, Patrick Chauvel and Renzo Guerrini. Published by Cambridge University Press. © Hermann Stefan, Elinor Ben-Menachem, Patrick Chauvel and Renzo Guerrini 2012.

Suggested reading

Canadian Clobazam Cooperative
Group. Clobazam in treatment of
refractory epilepsy: the Canadian
experience. *A retrospective study.*
Epilepsia; 1991; **32**: 407–16.

Glauser T, Ben-Menachem E,
Bourgeois B, *et al.* ILAE treatment
guidelines: evidence-based analysis
of antiepileptic drug efficacy and
effectiveness as initial
monotherapy for epileptic seizures
and syndromes. *Epilepsia* 2006; **4**:
1094–120.

Panayiotopoulos CP. Treatment of
typical absence seizures and related
epileptic syndromes. *Paediatr Drugs*
2001; **3**: 379–403.

Case

46

Episodic aphasia – surgery or not ?

Thilo Hammen and Hermann Stefan

Clinical history

A 51-year-old woman came to the epilepsy ambulance because of intractable seizures. Since the age of about 40 years she has suffered from simple focal, complex focal, and secondary tonic–clonic seizures. The patient reported aphasic dysfunction in which she is not able to think or speak sentences to the end. In addition, her husband complains about complex focal seizures with gazing, no reaction to speech and her environment, pausing and nestling mainly with the left hand. Duration: 3–4 minutes, frequency: once in 2 months. Secondary tonic–clonic seizures with tongue bite, opened eyes, and postictal sleep. Frequency: twice a year.

Examination

The right-handed patient suffers from decline of verbal memory; furthermore, regular findings in clinical neurological examination.

Neurological scores

Normal.

Special studies

Sleep-deprivation-EEG: inconstant theta-focus left temporal, no further pathological findings, particularly no findings of epileptic discharges.

Cranial MRI

Temporo-basal left popcorn-like lesion with a hemosiderin fringe (Fig. 1). The findings are consistent with a cavernous hemangioma.
    Routine laboratory tests: unremarkable.

Follow-up

The patient was scheduled for preoperative diagnostics in our epilepsy center. The patient declined further preoperative diagnosis because she was afraid of epilepsy surgery. Conservative therapy was started with oxcarbazepine and levetiracetam under which a reduction of seizure frequency and time duration of seizures was achieved. She was not seizure free under conservative treatment.

Diagnosis

Symptomatic epilepsy with simple focal, complex focal, and tonic–clonic seizures.

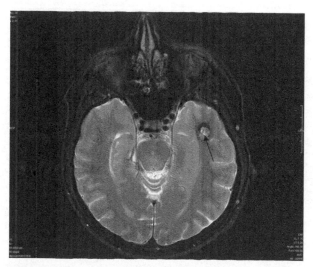

Fig. 1. Horizontal T2 weighted imaging demonstrating a temporo-basal left popcorn-like lesion with a hemosiderin fringe.

Case Studies in Epilepsy, ed. Hermann Stefan, Elinor Ben-Menachem, Patrick Chauvel and Renzo Guerrini. Published by Cambridge University Press. © Hermann Stefan, Elinor Ben-Menachem, Patrick Chauvel and Renzo Guerrini 2012.

General remarks

Supratentorial cavernous hemangiomas are often associated with symptomatic epilepsy. It is the aim of surgical treatment to control epilepsy and eliminate potential sources of intracerebral hematomas. Studies show that early surgical treatment of supratentorial cavernous hemangiomas provides better seizure outcome regardless of size or localization of cavernous hemangiomas (Stefan *et al.*, 2004).

Special remarks

Too often, patients are not operated on because patients and physicians are too cautious to start preoperative analysis. In most cases patients with epileptic cavernous hemangiomas turn out to be drug resistant in the course of the disease, as is our patient who still suffers from epileptic seizures.

Suggested reading

Smith K, Phoenix timing of surgical resection of cavernous malformation and seizure outcome. Poster 05.168, 62nd Annual Meeting of American Academy of Neurology, Toronto, 2010.

Stefan H, Walter J, Kerling F, Bluemcke I, Buchfelder M. Supratentorial cavernoma and epileptic seizures: predictors in postoperative control? *Der Nervenarzt* 2004; 75: 755–62.

Temporal lobe epilepsy: drugs or surgery?

Christophe Rauch and Hermann Stefan

History

A 37-year-old man has suffered from epilepsy since the age of 16. He reported simple partial seizures with an epigastric aura. His family reported seizures with staring, oral automatisms, and automatic movements of the hands. Rarely, there are generalized tonic–clonic seizures. At the age of three he had febrile convulsions. The rest of the medical history was unremarkable. He complained of about 3–4 seizures per month.

Actual treatment

Lamotrigine and levetiracetam in sufficient dosages.

Former antiepileptic treatment with carbamazepine and valproic acid.

What to do?
Further investigations

1. **MRI:** signs of hippocampus sclerosis right.
2. **Video–EEG:** interictal activity right temporomesial, ictal activity with seizure pattern right temporomesial.
3. **Neuropsychological assessment:** deficits in figural memory.

Diagnosis

Pharmacoresistant mesial temporal lobe epilepsy (MTLE) right.

Treatment

The patient was recommended for epilepsy surgery for a tailored resection right temporal.

General remarks

The patient has been seizure free since epilepsy surgery, but is still taking antiepileptic drugs. A pharmacoresistant epilepsy consists of pharmacotherapy with at least two different antiepileptic drugs in sufficient dosage.

Patients with the biggest chances of becoming seizure free after epilepsy surgery have symptomatic temporal lobe epilepsy with concordant results in MRI (e.g., hippocampus sclerosis), video–EEG monitoring, and neuropsychological assessment.

Special remarks

A particular cohort of patients with MTLE benefits most from surgical treatment. These are patients with very early initial precipitating injuries, a period of about 5 years without seizures, unequivocal unilateral EEG localization, MRI signs of mesial temporal sclerosis, and with contralateral memory compensation and ipsilateral reduced memory capacity shown in the neuropsychological investigation.

Suggested reading

Stefan H, Hildebrand M, Kerling F, *et al.* Clinical prediction of postoperative seizure control: structural, functional findings and disease histories. *J Neurol Neurosurg Psychiatry* 2009; **80:** 196–200.

Kwan P, Arzimanoglou A, Berg AT, Brodie MJ, *et al.* Definition of drug resistant epilepsy: consensus proposal by the ad hoc Task Force of the ILAE Commission on Therapeutic Strategies; *Epilepsia* 2010; **51:** 1069–77.

Case Studies in Epilepsy, ed. Hermann Stefan, Elinor Ben-Menachem, Patrick Chauvel and Renzo Guerrini. Published by Cambridge University Press. © Hermann Stefan, Elinor Ben-Menachem, Patrick Chauvel and Renzo Guerrini 2012.

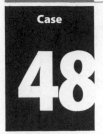

Case

48 Shaking in elderly: reversible or fate?

Christophe Rauch and Hermann Stefan

History

A 64-year-old man with a symptomatic focal epilepsy came to the outpatient service. He said he was seizure free under medication with valproic acid and lamotrigine. He complained of increasing memory problems, dizziness, and gait disorders.

Parkinson's disease was diagnosed due to psychomotoric slowing, body tremor, bradykinesia, and ataxia.

Actual treatment

Valproic acid 1500–0–1500 mg
Lamotrigine 150–0–150 mg
Madopar 62.5–0–62.5 mg

What to do?

Further investigations:

1. EEG: background activity 5–7/s, paroxysms 3/s delta waves, no epileptiform activity
2. Blood samples: serum concentrations
3. Valproic acid 135 µg/ml (normal: 50–100 µg/ml)
4. Lamotrigine 20 µg/ml (normal: 4–12 µg/ml)
5. NH_3 129 g/dl (normal 19–82 g/dl)

Diagnosis

Valproate-induced encephalopathy.

Treatment

The valproate dosage was reduced. The patient's physical and cognitive condition improved significantly. The EEG showed normalization of background activity.

General remarks

Valproate can cause an encephalopathy with symptoms that imitate Parkinson's disease with tremor and hypokinesia. This can occur, although valproate is well tolerated over years, so, it is important that these valproate-induced symptoms are not mistaken for a neurodegenerative disease. Compared with idiopathic parkinsonism, symptoms induced by valproate are usually reversible and can be resolved by withdrawal of the drug.

Special remarks

An overdosage of valproate can also lead to hyperammonemia, which causes deficits in cerebral energy metabolism, therefore, ammonia concentrations should be controlled in cases of suspected valproate-induced encephalopathy.

Suggested reading

Armon C, Shin C, Miller P, *et al.* Reversible parkinsonism and cognitive impairment with chronic valproate use. *Neurology* 1996; **47**: 626–35.

Göbel R, Görtzen A, Bräunig P. Enzephalopathien durch Valproat. *Fortschr Neurol Psychiatr* 1999; **67**: 7–11.

Masmoudi K, Gras-Champel V, Masson H, Andréjak M. Parkinsonism and/or cognitive impairment with valproic acid therapy: a report of 10 cases. *Pharmacopsychiatry* 2006; **39**: 9–12.

Onofrj M, Thomas A, Paci C. Reversible parkinsonism induced by prolonged treatment with valproate. *J Neurol* 1998; **245**: 794–6.

Case Studies in Epilepsy, ed. Hermann Stefan, Elinor Ben-Menachem, Patrick Chauvel and Renzo Guerrini. Published by Cambridge University Press. © Hermann Stefan, Elinor Ben-Menachem, Patrick Chauvel and Renzo Guerrini 2012.

Case

49

Failure of surgical treatment in a typical medial temporal lobe epilepsy

Jean-Pierre Vignal, Louis Maillard, Anne Thiriaux, and Sophie Colnat-Coulbois

History

In 2001, a 31-year-old right-handed woman was referred for presurgical evaluation of medically intractable epilepsy. At the age of 4 months, she had had prolonged febrile convulsions. Her first non-febrile seizures occurred at 21 years. Usually, seizures comprised an initial ascending epigastric sensation followed by a loss of contact, elementary gestural, and oro-alimentary automatisms. She had never had secondary generalizations. Interictal EEGs showed isolated right anterior temporal spikes. Partial seizures occurred 5–10 times per month. She reported occasional falls.

Seizures recorded during the long-term video–EEG monitoring had the following features: initial epigastric sensation, loss of contact, chewing automatisms, elementary gestural automatisms.

The patient had no other medical history and a normal neurological examination.

Investigations (2001)

Interictal EEG showed right temporal focal theta activity and rare right anterior temporal spikes. Three seizures were recorded: the first one lasted 120 seconds. She started to breath loudly, put down her book and warned: "I'm going to feel dizzy." She could initially carry out the instructions of the epilepsy nurse and had a face flush. Twenty seconds later, there was a loss of contact, chewing, and licking automatisms. She also had a right upper limb automatism of cranking and manipulating. Forty seconds after onset, she had a right head and eyes deviation. Postictal examination showed a transient confusion without any language disturbances (normal reading, naming, and understanding). She also retro-spectively gave a description of her initial epigastric

sensation. First modifications on EEG were detected 25 seconds after her warning and consisted of a right anterior temporal rhythmic theta (5 c/s) discharge, accelerating in 20 seconds to a more widespread right temporal spikes discharge (8 c/s), propagating to left temporal and right supra-sylvian electrodes. Postictal EEG showed a more pronounced right temporal slow activity and more frequent right temporal spikes.

The second seizure lasted 1 minute. The patient remained warned, remained fully aware and inter-acted during the whole course of the seizure. She described an epigastric sensation and seemed to be alarmed. There was no language disturbance. Ictal SPECT injection was performed within 10 seconds after onset. Ictal EEG showed a slow delta–theta right anterior temporal discharge.

The third seizure was identical to the first one.

MRI showed a right hippocampal sclerosis (HS). Interictal SPECT showed a right anterior temporal hypoperfusion. Ictal SPECT showed an increased per-fusion of the right temporal pole and temporo-medial structures.

Phase 1 synthesis

Initial epigastric sensation, chewing, gestural automa-tism, right anterior temporal theta, then spikes dis-charge and right temporal hyperperfusion on ictal SPECT support a right anterior medial temporal origin of seizures. Medical history and cranial MRI strongly support the responsibility of the right HS in generating these medial temporal lobe seizures (French et al., 1993; Williamson et al., 1993; Risinger et al., 1989).

Surgery

Based on these consistent data, a right anterior tem-poral partial lobectomy was carried out in 2001 (Fig 1).

Case Studies in Epilepsy, ed. Hermann Stefan, Elinor Ben-Menachem, Patrick Chauvel and Renzo Guerrini. Published by Cambridge University Press. © Hermann Stefan, Elinor Ben-Menachem, Patrick Chauvel and Renzo Guerrini 2012.

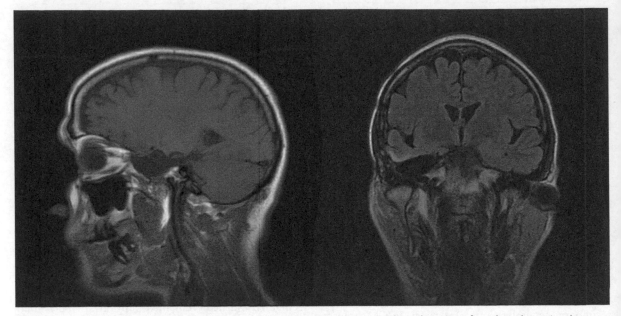

Fig. 1. Anterior medial temporal resection. The extent of lateral neocortical resection is limited to 4.5 cm from the pole, sparing the superior temporal gyrus. Resection of the amygdala, hippocampus and parahippocampus is performed.

It removed the right temporal pole, amygdala, anterior hippocampus, anterior basal temporal gyri, with the inferior temporal sulcus as a lateral limit. Treatment was immediately tapered. The patient was discharged from the neurosurgery department under a monotherapy of sodium valproate (1500 mg/day).

Postsurgical follow-up

Six months after the operation, she had a nocturnal generalized tonic–clonic seizure after having forgotten her AE treatment combined with sleep deprivation. Three years later, sodium valproate was replaced by carbamazepine (1200 mg/day) because of leukopenia.

Four years later (2005), she had two secondary generalized seizures preceded by an epigastric sensation. The re-occurrence of seizures was interpreted as secondary to an iatrogenic hyponatremia (126 millieq/l). Carbamazepine was replaced by levetiracetam (2000 mg/day). Five years after surgery (2006), she presented again with two secondary generalized tonic–clonic seizures initiated by an epigastric sensation. Levetiracetam was increased to 3000 mg/day. After a seizure-free interval of 1 year, she started having 1–2 partial seizures/month characterized by an initial epigastric sensation without any secondary generalization. Seizure frequency increased to 4–6 per month in 2009, despite an AE bitherapy. The seizures semiology could be limited to an isolated epigastric sensation (identical to the initial sensation reported before the operation) or comprised a loss of contact, right upper limb automatisms, and oro-alimentary automatisms.

New phase 1 (2009)

Interictal EEG showed a right temporal focal theta and spiking activity. Out of four recorded seizures, three comprised only an isolated sensation without any ictal EEG modification. Two possible anatomical origins were discussed for the remaining seizures: (i) an origin in the vicinity of the surgical resection (right posterior parahippocampal gyrus, basal, or lateral temporal gyri); (ii) a right insular origin. These conclusions prompted a depth-EEG investigation after discussing with the patient a possible second surgical resection.

Stereo-electroencephalography (SEEG) (2010)

Eight electrodes were implanted into the right hemisphere with the following targets:

_T: anterior superior temporal gyrus (STG)
_H: posterior insula (internal contacts) and posterior STG
_P: posterior cingulate gyrus–gyrus supra-marginalis

_TM: parahippocampal gyrus (internal contacts) – inferior temporal gyrus (ITG)

_F: posterior fusiform gyrus (internal contacts) – ITG (external contacts)

_B: posterior insula (internal contact) – posterior part of the middle temporal gyrus (MTG)

_O: anterior cingulate gyrus (internal contact) – inferior frontal gyrus (IFG, external contact)

_R: anterior insula (internal contacts) – IFG

Two electrodes were implanted in the left hemisphere:

_B': anterior hippocampus – MTG

_TB': peri-rhinal cortex – collateral sulcus – ITG

The understanding of this epilepsy relied upon the analysis of five spontaneous seizures and the results of cortical electrical stimulations. Four seizures occurred during wakefulness and one during nocturnal sleep. Anatomo-electro-clinical organization of all five seizures was identical. Ictal discharge started in the posterior insula (H, internal contacts), rapidly involved the whole insular cortex (B and R, internal contacts) and secondarily spread to the STG, frontal operculum and anterior cingulate cortex (Fig. 2). The patient reported an initial epigastric sensation three times when the discharge was confined in the right insula and once during postictal state.

Electrical stimulation of right posterior cingulated gyrus, right posterior and anterior-superior insula, right temporal operculum, left hippocampus, and left perirhinal cortex elicited an epigastric sensation identical to the earliest ictal symptom.

Case discussion

This case raises three issues for discussion.

The first is the diagnosis difficulty of the so-called "medial temporal epilepsy": indeed, in this patient all the features of the so-called medial temporal lobe epilepsy associated with hippocampal sclerosis were present (Najm et al., 2001). But the resection of the medial temporal structures did not cure the patient

on a long-term basis and the postsurgical ictal semiology was very close to the previous seizures observed prior to surgery: epigastric sensation, chewing, elementary gestural automatisms. The current observation emphasizes that a typical tableau of medial temporal lobe epilepsy after phase 1 investigations cannot exclude the possibility of an insular involvement in the epileptogenic zone, which can only be assessed by SEEG recordings. This insular involvement may explain part of the failures after anterior temporal lobectomy (Isnard and Mauguière, 2005) and illustrates the limitation of the concept of so-called medial temporal lobe epilepsy.

The second issue is the ubiquity of epigastric sensation (ES) as an ictal sign. ESs are frequent during temporal lobe seizures and often reflect the initial involvement of medial temporal structures (French et al., 1993; Maillard et al., 2004). However, abdominal auras are also reported in frontal lobe seizures (Williamson et al., 1985) and can be elicited by electrical stimulation of several cortical regions including limbic structures, opercular and insular cortices, and several frontal areas (Penfield and Faulk, 1955; Ostrowsky et al., 2000). In the current case, this symptom could be evoked by stimulation of different structures even outside the epileptogenic zone. In our case, the occurrence of ES during seizure reflected a local insular or temporo-limbic disturbance within a more widespread network involving both these structures and, most probably, related subcortical areas. The first surgery, which resected the temporal limbic structures, efficiently interrupted this network for several years, but this symptom re-appeared in relation with a localized insular discharge.

The third point is to emphasize the necessity of a long-term follow-up to assess the efficacy of surgical treatment for medically intractable partial epilepsies: indeed, in our case there is a gap of 7 years between surgery and recurrence of a medically intractable partial epilepsy.

Suggested reading

French JA, Williamson PD, Thadani VM, et al. Characteristics of medial temporal lobe epilepsy: I. Results of history and physical examination. Ann Neurol 1993; 34: 774–80.

Isnard J, Mauguière F. The insula in partial epilepsy. Rev Neurol (Paris) 2005; 161: 17–26.

Maillard L, Vignal JP, Gavaret M, et al. Semiologic and electrophysiologic correlations in temporal lobe seizure subtypes. Epilepsia 2004; 45: 1590–9.

Najm IM, Babb TL, Mohamed A, et al. Mesial temporal lobe sclerosis. In HO Lüders, YG Comair, eds. Epilepsy Surgery. Philadelphia: Lippincott Williams & Wilkins, 2001, 95–103.

Ostrowsky K, Isnard J, Ryvlin P, et al. Functional mapping of the insular

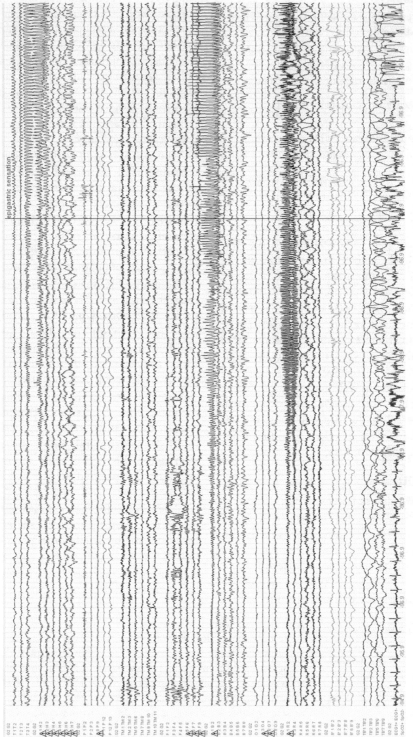

Fig. 2. EEG demonstrating right insular seizure onset. The seizure begins with high-frequency discharge (see the text for electrodes location).

cortex: clinical implication in temporal lobe epilepsy. *Epilepsia* *2000*; **41**: 681–6.

Penfield W, Faulk ME. The insula: further observations on its function. *Brain* 1955; **78**: 445–70.

Risinger MW, Engel J Jr, Van Ness PC, *et al.* Ictal localization of temporal lobe seizures wirth scalp/sphenoidal recordings. *Neurology* 1989; **39**: 1288–93.

Williamson PD, French JA, Thadani VM, *et al.* Characteristics of medial temporal lobe epilepsy: II. Interictal and ictal electroencephalography, neuropsychological testing, neuroimaging, surgical results, and pathology. *Ann Neurol* 1993; **34**: 781–7.

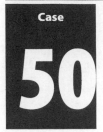

Case

50

Cutaneous adverse reactions by AEDs: chance or predetermination?

Xintong Wu and Hermann Stefan

Clinical history

A 28-year-old female with a history of epilepsy for almost 1 year (average one seizure per month), and a diagnosis of complex partial seizure was made by an epileptologist. She had taken per-oral carbamazepine for 5 days with a dosage of 100 mg three times a day. On presentation to the outpatient clinic of the neurology department, she had dermato-allergic reactions.

General history

She was an office worker who denied any previous use of alcohol, illicit drugs, or tobacco and any known previous drug allergies.

Examination

She had a temperature of 38.6 °c. Multiple maculopapule rashes were found all over the patient's face, trunk, and limbs (Fig. 1). Some blisters were found

(a)

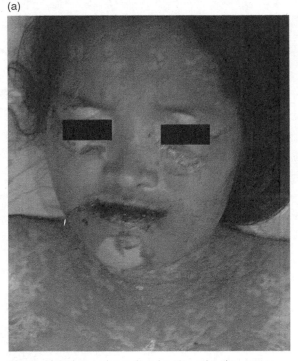

(b)

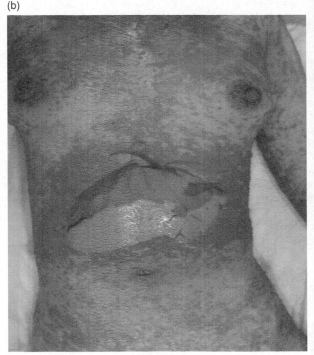

Fig. 1. Multiple maculopapule rashes. See color plate section.

Case Studies in Epilepsy, ed. Hermann Stefan, Elinor Ben-Menachem, Patrick Chauvel and Renzo Guerrini. Published by Cambridge University Press. © Hermann Stefan, Elinor Ben-Menachem, Patrick Chauvel and Renzo Guerrini 2012.

accompanied by rupture on face and trunk. Oral ulcers and hyperemic conjunctivae were also observed. Neurological examination was normal.

Follow-up

Considering hypersensitive reaction to carbamazepine to be its characteristic side effect, it was withdrawn immediately. The patient was then transferred to the dermatology department for diagnosis and treatment.

After admission to the dermatology department, the patient suffered a bad course of disease: the maculopapules mixed together gradually; more and more blisters appeared and ruptured in succession; the skin peeled away on some areas of the body surface; the lips and oral mucosa were involved and some ulcers occurred; the conjunctival hyperemia became more severe. She had a series of blood examinations and a skin biopsy.

Steroid, antihistamine, and γ-globulin and another adjuvant therapy were given to the patient. No AEDs were prescribed, considering the acute phase of allergic drug reaction. After effective treatment for several days, the patient had almost recovered and was discharged in a stable condition without sequelae. Then levetiracetam (500 mg twice a day) was used for seizure control.

Laboratory examination

No significant abnormal results of routine blood test (complete blood count and serum chemistries). C-reactive protein was 11.2 mg/l (reference range: < 5 mg/l).

The skin biopsy showed epidermal cell necrosis with some dyskeratotic keratinocytes and predominant lymphohistiocytic infiltration around the blood vessels and scanty eosinophils in dermis.

Diagnosis

1. Toxic epidermal necrolysis (TEN)
2. Complex partial seizure

General remarks

Antiepileptic drugs (AEDs) are one of the most common causes of cutaneous adverse drug reactions (cADRs), especially the aromatic compounds, including carbamazepine (CBZ), phenytoin (PHT), lamotrigine (LTG), oxcarbazepine (OXC) and phenobarbital (PB).

cADRs vary from mild maculopapular eruption (MPE), with increasing severity, to Stevens–Johnson syndrome (SJS), and toxic epidermal necrolysis (TEN).

SJS/TEN typically involves the skin and the mucous membranes. Oral, nasal, eye, vaginal, urethral, gastrointestinal, and lower respiratory tract mucous membranes may develop in the course of the illness.

SJS and TEN can be classified by the percentage of skin involved. SJS was defined as skin detachment of 10% of body-surface area or less; TEN was defined by skin detachment of 30% or more, whereas intermediate extent of skin detachment corresponded to SJS/TEN overlap. cADRs can also be accompanied with other symptoms and signs: fever, lymphadenopathy, hematological abnormalities, and involvement of at least one internal organ, for example, myocarditis, pneumonitis, nephritis and others. SJS and TEN are life-threatening severe cutaneous adverse drug reactions, with a mortality rate that can reach up to 40%.

cADRs are generally considered idiosyncratic. The pathogenesis of cADRs appears to be multifactorial and has in many cases been explained by the hapten hypothesis of drug hypersensitivity, which implies both metabolic and immunological mechanisms.

Special remarks

Some researchers suggest that genetic factors, rather than environmental factors, may be the reason for patients acquiring risks of AEDs-induced SJS/TEN.

As a strong association has been found between CBZ-induced SJS/TEN and HLA-B*1502, more and more researchers have investigated different alleles in AEDs-induced SJS/TEN. Up until now, the consensus has been that individuals who carry the HLA-B*1502 allele of the human leukocyte antigen gene may be more likely to develop severe skin conditions. This particular variant occurs predominantly in Asian populations. In Caucasians, based on insufficient evidence, no definitive conclusion has been obtained. The FDA has advised physicians to test Asian patients for the HLA-B*1502 allele prior to prescribing carbamazepine and to consider the potential risk of skin reactions when deciding whether to prescribe other aromatic AEDs. Additionally, other HLA alleles in different populations are still being investigated.

Once a patient has an allergic skin reaction to any one of the aromatic AEDs, other similar aromatic compounds should not be recommended. In order to control seizure, non-aromatic AEDs, such as valproic acid, topiramate, levetiracetam, etc. can be considered.

Suggested reading

Alfirevic A, Jorgensen AL, Williamson PR, *et al.* HLA-B locus in Caucasian patients with carbamazepine hypersensitivity. *Pharmacogenomics* 2006; **7**: 813–18.

Chung WH, Hung SI, Hong HS, *et al.* Medical genetics: a marker for Stevens–Johnson syndrome. *Nature* 2004; **428**: 486.

Chung WH, Hung SI, Chen YT. Genetic predisposition of life-threatening antiepileptic-induced skin reactions. *Expert Opin Drug Saf* 2010; **9**: 15–21.

Ferrell PB Jr, McLeod HL. Carbamazepine, HLA-B*1502 and risk of Stevens-Johnson syndrome and toxic epidermal necrolysis: US FDA recommendations. *Pharmacogenomics* 2008; **9**: 1543–6.

Lonjou C, Thomas L, Borot N, *et al.* A marker for Stevens–Johnson syndrome – ethnicity matters. *Pharmacogenomics J* 2006; **6**: 265–8.

Man CB, Kwan P, Baum L, *et al.* Association between HLA-B*1502 allele and antiepileptic drug-induced cutaneous reactions (in Han Chinese). *Epilepsia* 2007; **48**: 1015–18.

Messenheimer J, Mockenhaupt M, Tennis P, *et al.* Incidence of Stevens–Johnson syndrome and toxic epidermal necrolysis among new users of antiepileptic drugs. *Neurology* 2004; **62**: S41.

Roujeau JC. The spectrum of Stevens–Johnson syndrome and toxic epidermal necrolysis: a clinical classification. *J Invest Dermatol* 1994; **102**: 28S–30S.

Svensson CK, Cowen EW, Gaspari AA. Cutaneous drug reactions. *Pharmacol Rev.* 2000; **53**: 357–79.

Toledano R and Gil-Nagel A. Adverse effects of antiepileptic drugs. *Semin Neurol* 2008; **28**: 317–27.

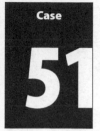

Case

51

Timing of medical and surgical treatment of epilepsy: a hemispherotomy that would have prevented disabling cerebellar atrophy

Jörg Wellmer

Clinical history

A 25-year-old male patient presented to our outpatient clinic with a medical history of seizure onset at the age of 12 and up to 170 seizures per day despite anticonvulsive treatment. Due to long-standing phenytoin overdosage he had developed severe cerebellar atrophy, lost fine motor skills and was confined to a wheelchair. Because of obviously unilateral, non-dominant seizure onset, an earlier right hemispherotomy could have stopped seizures and – at the cost of left hemiplegia – might have prevented the disabling ataxia. This case illustrates the difficulties of choosing the right point in time for medical and surgical epilepsy treatment.

Medical history

After a regular pregnancy and birth the male patient had had an uneventful cognitive and motor development until the age of 12. At that age, after a horse-riding lesson, he experienced an episode of dizziness, gait instability and confusion lasting several minutes, followed by tingling paresthesias in the left part of his body. This episode was repeated twice the next day. He was admitted to a children's hospital where the physical examination was normal. MRI revealed an edematous swelling in the right anterior cerebral artery territory, the right insula, and the right hippocampus – no further pathologies were described. Copies of the initial MRI are no longer available. This disseminated lesion pattern was interpreted as multifocal ischemia. A familiar hyperlipoproteinemia type A was suspected to be the cause since no other predisposing conditions for ischemia were identified.

Between the episodes and over the following 2 months, the patient still had no neurological deficit.

He was able to play football with his mates. Two months later he developed left-sided clonic seizures, up to 170 per day.

History of anticonvulsive treatment

Over the following years the patient was seen by several pediatric and epilepsy clinics. In various combinations he was prescribed carbamazepine, oxcarbazepine, lamotrigine, mesuximide, phenobarbital, phenytoin, sultiam, topiramate, valproic acid, and vigabatrin. None of these substances led to a substantial reduction of the seizure frequency. A vagal nerve stimulator (VNS) was implanted without effect on the seizure frequency. Phenytoin was understood to be the basic treatment since every attempt at reduction led to a series of seizures and statuses, which often had to be terminated by intensive care treatment. Over time, the phenytoin dose was successively increased. The highest documented phenytoin blood level was 90 µg/ml (normal range: 5–20, toxic effects above 25 µg/ml). According to medical reports, except for VNS, at no time point was an alternative to pharmaceutical treatment discussed.

At presentation, the daily medication comprised 500 mg phenytoin (serum concentration 70 µg/ml), levetiracetam 6000 mg, and phenobarbital 100 mg. The current seizure frequency was 10–15 per day.

Physical history

With each status epilepticus over the first years of epilepsy, remission of postictal left-sided motor deficits became more incomplete. One year after onset, he required a wheelchair for longer distances. Nystagm, dysarthrophonia, and ataxia developed gradually. At 16, walking was possible only with support,

Case Studies in Epilepsy, ed. Hermann Stefan, Elinor Ben-Menachem, Patrick Chauvel and Renzo Guerrini. Published by Cambridge University Press. © Hermann Stefan, Elinor Ben-Menachem, Patrick Chauvel and Renzo Guerrini 2012.

and handwriting became unreadable. Yet, with his right arm he was still able to perform skills such as eating. Even these fine motor skills got lost over time. Five years after the onset of seizures and anticonvulsive therapy, he was dysarthric. Bradydisdiadochokinesis was documented for the right hand. Gait was impossible due to lack of trunk control. Phenytoin overdosage was already documented ("after tapering 34.1 µg/ml"). The patient had gingival hyperplasia.

Social history

At the age of 16, he had to be taken away from school. He was referred to day-time support in a sheltered workshop.

Examination at outpatient clinic presentation

At presentation in our clinic, the patient was bound to an electric wheelchair. He showed a moderate non-spastic 2/5 hemiparesis of the left arm and leg. Dystonic left hand and arm (no contracture). Left central facial palsy. Right arm and leg formally without paresis, but held dystonically, severe ataxia. No fine motor skills possible. Gait possible only with support – highly atactic. Tendon reflexes of legs bilaterally weak, left arm difficult to estimate because of dystonic position, but not pronounced compared to the right arm. No pyramidal signs. Reduced sensibility of the left half of the body. Initiation of movement and speech markedly slowed. High-grade dysarthrophonia and motility disturbance of the tongue, including disturbance of swallowing. Irregular fixation nystagm and end position nystagmus. Cognitively slowed but awake, oriented. No obvious cognitive impairment. Massive gingival hyperplasia (Fig. 1).

Seizure semiology

Three years after seizure onset: type 1: contracture followed by rhythmic cloni of the left corner of the mouth, then smacking, hypersalivation. No loss of consciousness. type 2: starting as type 1, then propagation of tonic activity to the whole left half of the body, later clonic phase. Occasionally, bilateral propagation. Frequency at admission to a hospital: with intervals of 10–20 minutes nearly continuous during wake and sleep. No seizure-free day since 2 years.

Current semiology – Type 1: eyes wide open, starring, loss of reagibility, grimacing. Duration: few

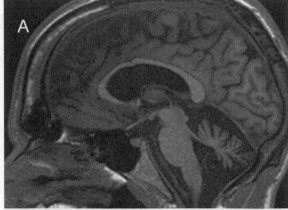

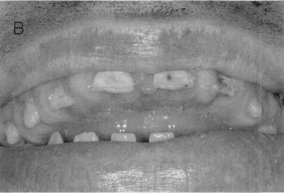

Fig. 1. (a) Magnetic resonance imaging demonstrates severe cerebellar atrophy as consequence of long-standing phenytoin over dosage. Highest documented phenytoin blood levels were 70 µg/ml. (b) Photograph of the massive gingival hyperplasia as common side effect of phenytoin intake.

seconds. Formally 10–15/day, at present no type 1 seizure. Type 2: starting as type 1 but followed by hypersalivation, contraction of the left corner of the mouth, tonic then clonic elevation of the left arm, vocalization. Duration: 30 seconds. 1/day. Type 3: Starting as type 1 and 2, then secondary generalization, often in series with intervals of 5 minutes. Last generalized seizure 6 months ago.

Treatment plan

Knowing about statuses after earlier attempts to taper phenytoin, but also realizing the need to reduce phenytoin to prevent further progression of cerebellar atrophy, we intended to work out if hemispherotomy was an option to stop the seizures and be able to reduce the AED load. A retrospective evaluation of previous reports indicated that obviously all recorded interictal discharges had a right hemispheric origin.

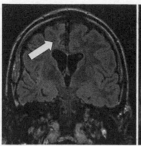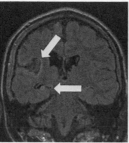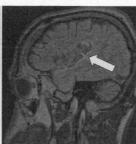

Fig. 2. Magnetic resonance imaging demonstrating the defect zones distributed over the right hemisphere: right fronto-mesial cortex, right insula cortex, right hippocampal sclerosis, right hemiatrophia. The left hemisphere is unaffected.

Also, seizures were recorded only with right hemispheric rhythmic activity.

At current physical examination, the left side of the body was not functional, so that quality of life would not be worsened by a fixed left hemiplegia. We rather expected to improve his quality of life by a reduction of the permanent intoxication with phenytoin.

Inpatient examination

A video EEG monitoring revealed that seizures under tapering phenytoin (over 100 seizures recorded in 2 days – types 2 and 3 of the current semiology) originated from the right hemisphere. Interictal epileptic discharges were very frequent, at times nearly continuous. The clear focus was over the right hemisphere; only a few interictal discharges were also registered from left frontal.

MRI under narcosis showed right hemispheric hemiatrophy, cortical defect in parts of the right ACA territory, right insula and right hippocampal sclerosis (Fig. 2). We found no contralateral damage. As expected, MRI also revealed a severe bilateral cerebellar atrophy with maximum in the vermis (Fig. 1) (De Marcos *et al.*, 2003).

Hemispherotomy became more likely. To exclude partial right hemispheric language representation and to identify the left frontal interictal discharges as a result of secondary bilateral synchrony from the right, a unilateral right amobarbital WADA test was scheduled (Wellmer *et al.*, 2005). To rule out a mitochondrial defect, which could cause further harm to the patient after application of amobarbital (Niehusmann *et al.*, 2011), a mitochondrial diagnostic was performed. Tests for MELAS (A3243G, A8344G) and LHON (3460A, 11778A, 14459A, 14484C) were negative.

However, while waiting for the mitochondrial test results, we introduced lacosamide. This unexpectedly allowed tapering of phenytoin with only one short series of seizures. Finally, under co-medication with lacosamide, levetiracetam, and phenobarbital, phenytoin could be reduced to non-toxic levels of 15 μg/ml. Tapering of phenytoin resulted in an increased alertness and reduced the cognitive slowing. Under 3-week intensive physiotherapy and ergotherapy, the patient improved slightly with his right arm functionality. Yet, fine motor skills were still not possible (such as eating, drinking, tooth brushing). The patient was referred to a rehabilitation clinic. By this time, the patient had preliminarily decided against hemispherotomy because of an acceptable seizure situation and the expectation that there was no further benefit from surgery. Rehabilitation of 6 weeks did not lead to a further improvement of his fine motor skills, but he was taught to use a computer with a special keyboard and a mouse, which now allows him to take over some duties in his sheltered workshop.

General comments

This case report illustrates the problem of timing medical and surgical treatment of epilepsy patients. Without any doubt, the initial treatment of epileptic seizures is the domain of anticonvulsive drugs (Brodie and Kwan, 2002). If anticonvulsive treatment is successful, there should be no events that harm social development (school, professional education and occupation, marital status), despite the persisting predisposition for seizures. The risks of epilepsy-associated cognitive decline, morbidity, and mortality decreases with seizure control (Thompson and Duncan 2005; Sillanpää and Shinnar, 2010).

Yet, when initial anticonvulsive drug treatment fails, it is difficult to predict whether repeated modifications of drugs will eventually stop seizures. Etiology of seizures can give some hint on the likelihood of remission. Focal epilepsy is more likely to be pharmacoresistant than idiopathic generalized epilepsy, and among patients with focal epilepsy worse outcomes have been documented for patients with mesial temporal sclerosis and dysplastic lesions (Semah *et al.*, 2005). Yet, due to the large inter-individual variability of courses of the disease, individual prediction of response to medication is impossible.

Possibly because of a strong belief in late success of medication or because of a lack of familiarity with the efficacy and low morbidity of epilepsy surgery (Benbadis *et al.*, 2003), there is a tendency towards late referral of patients to specialized epilepsy units. Referral times of 20 years after the onset of seizures are not uncommon (Berg *et al.*, 2003; Benbadis *et al.*, 2003). Yet, too much hope in late medical success can have a negative impact on patients. Even studies arguing in favor of repeated modification of anticonvulsive drugs (such as those of Luciano and Shorvon (2007) and Callaghan *et al.* (2007)) demonstrate that the majority of patients with initial therapeutic failure remain pharmacoresistant even after multiple modifications.

Guidance in the decision for continued medical or surgical treatment comes from the definition of pharmacoresistance which was published by the ILAE Commission on Therapeutic Strategies (Kwan *et al.*, 2010). This report makes clear, that pharmacoresistance does not mean resistance of an individual against all available anticonvulsive drugs as the term might imply. They state that *any definition of drug resistance must be based on an assessment of the probability of subsequent remission after each drug failure.* According to the commission, pharmacoresistance may be defined as a *failure of adequate trials of two tolerated and appropriately chosen and used AED schedules* to avoid unnecessary delay in evaluation of alternative treatment options, which is in the first place epilepsy surgery. However, *because presurgical evaluation and surgery itself may entail risks, the decision to offer surgical treatment requires individual risk-benefit analysis* (Kwan *et al.*, 2010).

A first estimate of the individual risk–benefit ratio of epilepsy surgery is possible after a careful patient interview regarding his or her precise seizure semiology, a routine EEG and, most importantly, a high-quality MRI, which is evaluated by a radiologist or epileptologist with expertise in the evaluation of epilepsy MRIs. In the case of easily accessible and completely removable epileptogenic lesions that lie remote from eloquent cortex, the chance for postoperative seizure freedom can be up to 90% (Wagner *et al.*, 2011). In these cases definite presurgical work-up and epilepsy surgery should be offered to the patient after the second failed AED at the latest. Unnecessary delay in surgery may be more risky than the surgery itself. The worse the risk–benefit ratio (including the

need for complex invasive work-up), the more AED trials should be made before considering surgery. The MRI-based approach to "relative pharmacoresistance" has been described by Wellmer and Elger (2009).

However, it must be stressed that incorrect classification of patients as non-lesional, following suboptimal MRI quality or an inexperienced reader, will result in misclassifying as bad surgical candidates (von Oertzen *et al.*, 2002). Therefore, these classifications should be made by specialized epilepsy surgery units to which patients have to be referred.

Among all surgical procedures, hemispherotomy requires separate attention. Unless the patient already suffers from high-grade paresis and hemianopia contralateral to the intended surgery, these consequences of surgery have to be accepted as inevitable. There are still patients with severely disabling and harmful seizures (such as epileptic drop attacks) in whom hemiparesis and hemianopia are acceptable because of the chance of a cure cure after hemispherotomy. In well-selected cases, this chance is high (78%) (Limbrick *et al.*, 2009). Because of this high success rate, in some cases even the decision for de-afferentiation of the dominant hemisphere can be justified, particularly if a progressive disease will cause loss of language functions anyway. An example of this scenario is Rasmussen's encephalitis (Bien and Schramm, 2009). Nevertheless, surgery should be performed as early as possible. The younger children are at surgery, the more complete is the (re-) development of language (Vining *et al.*, 1997).

In the present case the right time window for hemispherotomy was missed. Seizures were unresponsive to medication from the beginning. Several attempts to modify the medication did not result in seizure control. An early MRI showed cortical defects distributed only throughout the right hemisphere. At the very beginning left motor function was not impaired, therefore, an early presurgical work-up would have correctly come to the conclusion that the risk–benefit ratio was on the side of continued medical treatment.

However, as time went on, there was increasing motor dysfunction of the left side, and because of the phenytoin intoxication the primarily non-affected right side of the body was also affected. At this stage it was predictable that continued high-level phenytoin would finally cause irreversible cerebellar atrophy. If, at that time, another presurgical assessment had been performed, the balance would have been on the side of surgery. Hemispherotomy would have been the surgery of choice, since it would have offered a realistic chance of seizure freedom at the cost of fixed hemiparesis and hemianopia, but the functionality of the right side of the body could have been preserved. The long-term quality of life of the patient would certainly have come out better than it is now.

Today, the risk–benefit ratio of medical and surgical treatment has changed again. Because of irreversible cerebellar atrophy, fine motor skills are lost, even in the formerly healthy right side of the body. On the other hand, under lacosamide in combination with phenytoin (at non-toxic levels), levetiracetam and phenobarbital, the seizure situation is acceptable with regard to his life circumstances (he is still confined to a wheelchair). Unless the seizure situation worsens again, hemispherotomy no longer makes sense.

Follow-up

1 year after originally writing this report the patient again worsened despite unchanged medication. He had series of seizures, which had to be terminated by narcotics. Pehytoin and Phenobarbital were elevated back to toxic levels to get him from ventilation. Video-EEG-monitoring at the intensive care unit again documented only right hemispheric seizure onset. A right hemispheric Wada text did not show any language impairment. Interictal bi-hemispheric epileptic activity ceased with the isolated right Wada test, proving spike propagation only from right to left. A functional hemispherotomy was performed. Since surgery (2 months) the patient is completely seizure free and phenytoin and Phenobarbital levels were at normal range.

Conclusions

What can be learned from this case is that, whenever during the course of epilepsy therapeutic decisions have to be made, alternative treatment options should be considered. If there is a chance of a cure by surgery, this should be seriously considered and offered to a patient. Perpetuated medical treatment is not automatically the less harmful option.

Suggested reading

Benbadis SR, Heriaud L, Tatum WO, Vale FL. Epilepsy surgery, delays and referral patterns – are all your epilepsy patients controlled? *Seizure* 2003; **12**: 167–70.

Berg AT, Vickrey BG, Langfitt JT, *et al*. Multicenter Study of Epilepsy Surgery. The multicenter study of epilepsy surgery: recruitment and selection for surgery. *Epilepsia* 2003; **44**: 1425–33.

Bien CG, Schramm J. Treatment of Rasmussen encephalitis half a century after its initial description: promising prospects and a dilemma. *Epilepsy Res* 2009; **86**: 101–12.

Brodie MJ, Kwan P. Staged approach to epilepsy management. *Neurology* 2002; **58**: S2–8.

Callaghan BC, Anand K, Hesdorffer D, Hauser WA, French JA. Likelihood of seizure remission in an adult population with refractory epilepsy. *Ann Neurol* 2007; **62**: 382–9.

De Marcos FA, Ghizoni E, Kobayashi E, Li LM, Cendes F. Cerebellar volume and long-term use of phenytoin. *Seizure* 2003; **12**: 312–15.

Kwan P, Arzimanoglou A, Berg AT, *et al*. Definition of drug resistant epilepsy: consensus proposal by the ad hoc Task Force of the ILAE Commission on Therapeutic Strategies. *Epilepsia* 2010; **51**: 1069–77.

Limbrick DD, Narayan P, Powers AK, *et al*. Hemispherotomy: efficacy and analysis of seizure recurrence. *J Neurosurg Pediatr* 2009; **4**: 323–32.

Luciano AL, Shorvon SD. Results of treatment changes in patients with apparently drug-resistant chronic epilepsy. *Ann Neurol* 2007; **62**: 375–81.

Niehusmann P, Surges R, von Wrede RD, *et al*. Mitochondrial dysfunction due to Leber's hereditary optic neuropathy as a cause of visual loss during assessment for epilepsy surgery. *Epilepsy Behav* 2011; **20**: 38–43.

Semah F, Ryvlin P. Can we predict refractory epilepsy at the time of diagnosis? *Epileptic Disord* 2005; **7**: S10–13.

Sillanpää M, Shinnar S. Long-term mortality in childhood-onset epilepsy. *N Engl J Med* 2010; **363**: 2522–9.

Thompson PJ, Duncan JS. Cognitive decline in severe intractable epilepsy. *Epilepsia* 2005; **46**: 1780–7.

Vining EP, Freeman JM, Pillas DJ, *et al*. Why would you remove half a brain? The outcome of 58 children after hemispherectomy – the Johns Hopkins experience: 1968 to 1996. *Pediatrics* 1997; **100**: 163–71.

Von Oertzen J, Urbach H, Jungbluth S, *et al*. Standard magnetic resonance imaging is inadequate for patients with refractory focal epilepsy. *J Neurol Neurosurg Psychiatry* 2002; **73**: 643–7.

Wagner J, Urbach H, Niehusmann P, *et al*. Focal cortical dysplasia type IIb: completeness of cortical, not subcortical, resection is necessary for seizure freedom. *Epilepsia* 2011; **52**: 1418–24.

Wellmer J, Elger CE. MRI in the presurgical evaluation. In S Shorvon, E Perucca, J Engel, eds. *The Treatment of Epilepsy*. Wiley-Blackwell, 2009, 805–20.

Wellmer J, Fernández G, Linke DB, *et al*. Unilateral intracarotid amobarbital procedure for language lateralization. *Epilepsia* 2005; **46**: 1764–72.

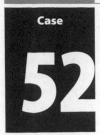

Anticonvulsive drugs for gait disturbance and slurred speech?

Hermann Stefan

Clinical history

In childhood, dizziness and falling. During these short attacks the (34-year-old today) patient became pale and suffered at the same time from hyperhidrosis, slurred speech, double vision horizontally. Sometimes, he had the impression that his mind was slowed. Duration of these signs was about 10 minutes, sometimes even hours, occurring several times per day. Sleep deprivation and alcohol were the precipitating triggers. In adolescence these paroxsmal signs spontaneously disappeared, but re-occurred at the age of 25 with a frequency of up to three to four times weekly. A sudden onset of clouding of consciousness without motoric or autonomic signs was reported.

Examination

Neurological findings: facial assymetry, horizontal nystagmus, bilateral hypacusis and a discrete hemispastic syndrome, dysdiadochokinesis, and pathological Romberg and Unterberger test.

Laboratory investigations showed no pathological findings, no inborn error of metabolism.

The EEG showed alpha background activity and during an attack 6/s generalized theta waves, no epileptiform potentials.

Imaging

The MRI displayed an atrophy of the cerebellar vermis.

Diagnosis

Episodic ataxia.

General remarks

For differential diagnosis, at first we have to note an episodic functional disorder with special predominant clinical signs pointing to the cerebellar and brainstem system. As leading sign a cerebellar ataxia and, in addition, dysarthria, vertigo and diplopia; furthermore nystagmus and autonomic signs were reported.

From family history we learn that several members of the family suffer from similar episodic attacks. Concerning differential diagnosis, one has to consider familiar episodic ataxia. Similar paroxysmal phenomena can occur within multiple sclerosis. Here we find paroxysmal bulbar dysarthria and severe ataxia for a short duration of seconds. Sometimes it is accompanied by disturbance of vision or paresthesia in the trigeminal area. The duration of the attacks starting in the patient's early childhood and familiar disposition would be unusual for multiple sclerosis.

Other subjective signs, such as slowing of mind, the "loss of consciousness" could be due to epileptic activity or syncopes, but no further findings could prove this suspicion.

Differential diagnosis could also consider transient visual disturbance in the vertebrobasilar territory, which also may cause drop attacks. During drop attacks patients promptly fall to the ground, but this was not the case with our patient, cerebral circulation was normal. Rarely, paroxysmal tonic upgaze is associated with ataxia. Episodic ataxia (EA) can be accompanied by a variety of other neurological signs. Six subtypes of episodic ataxias are differentiated. EA_1 only lasts for a few minutes. It is caused by missense point mutations of $KCNA_1$ and can be treated with CBZ (PHT). EA_2 attacks are prolonged. They may be provoked by exercise, stress, or alcohol. In the spell-free interval, central ocular

---

Case Studies in Epilepsy, ed. Hermann Stefan, Elinor Ben-Menachem, Patrick Chauvel and Renzo Guerrini. Published by Cambridge University Press. © Hermann Stefan, Elinor Ben-Menachem, Patrick Chauvel and Renzo Guerrini 2012.

motor dysfunction (predominantely down beat nystagmus) can exist. In addition to acetazolamide (70%), 4-amino pyramidine (K-channel blocker) was effective.

Special remarks

Episodic ataxias are also observed in inborn errors of metabolism such as hereditary hyperamm-onemia, hyperalaninemia or pyruvate dysmetabolism syndrome as well as in Hartnup disease. In these conditions severe neurological and psychic defects with recessive genetic trait were often observed.

Anticonvulsive treatment by means of carbamazepine and/or acetazolamide controlled the attacks.

Suggested reading

Andermann FJ, Cosgrove JB, Lloyd-Smith D, Walter AM. Paroxysmal dysarthria and ataxia in multiple sclerosis. A report of 2 unusual cases. *Neurology (Minneapolis)* 1959; **9**: 211–15.

Donat JR, Auger R. Acetazolamide in the treatment of pyruvate dysmetabolism syndromes. *Arch Neurol* 1978; **35**: 302–5.

Grigg R, Maxley RT, La France RA, *et al*. Hereditary paroxysmal ataxia: Response to acetazolamide. *Neurology (Minneapolis)* 1978; **28**: 1259–64.

Imbrici P, Jaffe SL, Eunson LH, *et al*. Dysfunction of the brain calcium channel CaV2.1 in absence epilepsy and episodic ataxia. 2004; **127**: 2682–92.

Lispi M, Vigivano F. Benign paroxysmal tonic upgaze fo childhood with ataxia. *Epileptic Disord* 2001; **3**: 203–6.

Wolf P. Familiäre episodische Ataxie. *Nervenarzt* 1980; **51**: 355–8.

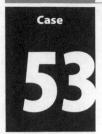

53

Unsuccessful surgery: another chance?

Hermann Stefan

General history

Since the age of 6, focal seizures, epigastric auras, tingling ascending from the stomach to the head, then into left arm and leg from proximal to distal into right arm and leg, acoustic hallucinations, hearing music, and incomprehensible voices. In addition, clouding of consciousness, stare gaze, oral and gesticulating automatisms, preserved speech, sometimes falling, and secondary convulsive seizures.

Treatment with carbamazepine, valproate, phenytoin, vigabatrin, clobazam, phenobarbital, levetiracetam, sultiam, and gabapentin as well as zonisamide without seizure control.

Family history

Father suffers from paranoid hallucinatory psychosis. No family history of epilepsy, febrile convulsion, head injuries, or other disease.

Clinical history

The patient underwent surgery by tailored resection temporal right, including anterior temporal neocortex and hippocampal resection.

Histological examination of the resected specimen showed dual pathology with hippocampal sclerosis and diffuse heterotopia. Postoperatively, seizure control was obtained for 8 weeks, then seizures reoccurred with a frequency of six focal seizures with secondary convulsions per months. Seizure duration turned out shorter than prior to surgery, but falling with injuries during seizures occurred again.

Re-evaluation of the 40-year-old female patient showed on MRI a resection volume due to the epilepsy surgery performed.

In the SPECT investigation, in addition to the missing radionuclide enhancement temporal right, temporal left hyperperfusion.

The neurological investigation showed quadrant anopsia to the left upright and increased memory problems as well as depression.

The anticonvulsant treatment was changed, but the patient reported dizziness, and headache after neurontin. Treatment with lamotrigine showed a positive effect on mood, but control on seizure activity could not be obtained.

Five years after first surgery a re-operation was discussed. The second epilepsy surgery was performed in a broad standard resection of neocortical and mesial structures. Re-operation turned out unsuccessful.

Examinations

Neurological findings: Normal. Right-handed. Slight memory impairment.

Because of pharmacoresistant epilepsy, the patient was referred to presurgical evaluation for epilepsy surgery.

EEG: Intermittent theta, slowing fronto temporal right as well as sharp waves, 82% right, 18% left.

During seizure onset, flattening rhythmic 7/s theta activity was recorded; temporal right with propagation to left.

Imaging

MRI shows hippocampal sclerosis.

Diagnosis

Pharmacoresistant TLE with two unsuccessful epilepsy surgeries.

Case Studies in Epilepsy, ed. Hermann Stefan, Elinor Ben-Menachem, Patrick Chauvel and Renzo Guerrini. Published by Cambridge University Press. © Hermann Stefan, Elinor Ben-Menachem, Patrick Chauvel and Renzo Guerrini 2012.

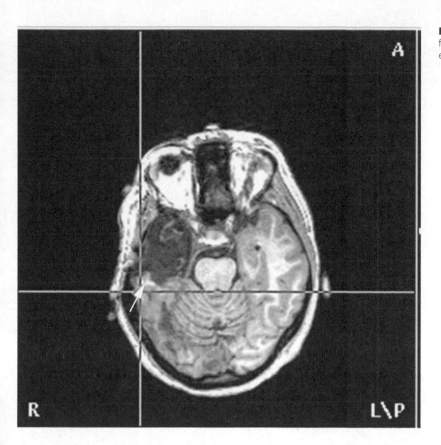

Fig. 1. Postoperative MEG. Remaining focal epileptic activity after two epilepsy surgeries.

Follow-up

Two years later simultaneous magnetoencephalography (MEG) and EEG recordings were performed. For the analysis, dipoles and a realistic head model were used. The source localizations were visualized with regard to the patient's anatomy using the individual MRI. The results showed focal epileptic activity (Fig. 1) because the patient still suffered from falling seizures and side effects of the anticonvulsive medication and was not willing to undergo any further invasive procedures. Focal radiation was discussed. Finally, stereotactic low-dose fractionated radiotherapy (Novalis system) was applied and the patient became seizure free. The radiation dose was 11×3 gy. No side effects were reported. MRI showed no further changes.

Meanwhile, the patient has been seizure free for 3 years.

General remarks

In addition to resective epilepsy surgery meanwhile, other treatment approaches are available, such as vagus nerve stimulation, deep brain stimulation, or radiosurgery/therapy. The patient was offered all treatment approaches and finally chose radiotherapy.

First reports about radiation in the treatment of epilepsies were by Tracy *et al.* (1905). In animal models, the effect of ionizing radiation on epileptic activity was demonstrated by Barcia-Salorio (1987) and Chen *et al.* (2001). Further investigations in humans using X-ray gamma knife surgery in mesial temporal lobe epilepsies were reposted by Regis *et al.* (1999).

Special remarks

Whereas in temporal lobe epilepsies, single short gamma knife radiosurgery in a considerable number of patients led to seizure control, radiotherapy using low-dose fractionated irradiation was used in patients who could not be operated on or who had been operated on unsuccessfully. Low-dose stereotactic fractionated radiotherapy aims to modulate epileptic activity without neuronal destruction in focal epilepsies with seizure onset in functional important areas. In contrast to gamma knife surgery in mesial temporal lobe epilepsies, up to now low dose focal radiotherapy has not been used in place of epilepsy surgery. It is only used as an ultima ratio or last resort.

Suggested reading

Barbaro NM, *et al.* A multicenter prospective pilot study of gamma knife radiosurgery for mesial temporal lobe epilepsy: seizure response, adverse events and verbal memory. *Ann Neurol* 2009; **65**: 167–75.

Barcia-Salorio JL, Vanalocha V, Cerdá M, Ciudad J, López-Gómez L. Response of experimental epileptic focus to focal ionizing radiation. *Appl Neurophysiol* 1987; **50**: 359–64.

Regis J, Semah F, Bryan RN, *et al.* Early and delayed MR and PET changes after selective temporomesial radiosurgery in mesial temporal lobe epilepsy. *AJNR Am J Neuroradiol* 1999; **20**: 213–16.

Stefan H, *et al.* Successful treatment of focal epilepsy by fractionated stereotactic radio therapy. *Eur Neurol* 1998; **39**: 248–50.

Tracy SG. High frequency high potential currents and X-radiation in the treatment of epilepsies. *N York MJ* 1905; **81**: 422–4.

Chen ZF, Toshifumi K, Scott LH, *et al.* Anticonvulsant effects of gamma surgery in a model of chronic spontaneous limbic epilepsy rats. *J Neurosurg* 2001; **94**: 270–80.

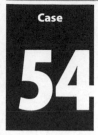

54

If it's not broken, don't fix it!

Elinor Ben-Menachem

This woman was born in 1969. At the age of five she developed absence epilepsy with three per second spike and wave activity on the EEG. She was given ethosuximide and was free of her absences after that. However, at the age of 13, she also started having generalized tonic–clonic seizures Phenytoin was added and she was again seizure free for 6 years, but the blood concentration of phenytoin hovered around 90 μmol/l. She graduated from high school and lived a normal life with the exception that she had some gingival hyperplasia and complained of being tired. In 1993 her physician thought that, because phenytoin is not a recommended drug for absence epilepsy, and because she had side effects from phenytoin in the form of gingival hyperplasia, he would switch her to valproate, which was the drug thought to be more effective for her epilepsy syndrome and does not cause gingival hyperplasia.

In 1994 phenytoin was slowly down-titrated and valproate started. She had a few tonic–clonic seizures during the switch after being seizure free for so many years. Then after 3 months, when she was in the process of switching (phenytoin blood concentration was 60 μmol/l), she came into the hospital in an ambulance with generalized status epilepticus. Her valproate dose at that time was 1800 mg/day. Phenytoin was, of course, restarted by intravenous infusion so that the blood concentration rapidly reached 120 μmol/l. She was given thiopental in the intensive care unit and finally the status stopped after 3 days.

After recovery, she was sent home with the combination of phenytoin, valproate, and ethosuximide. Unfortunately, she did not ever regain seizure freedom and not only suffered from generalized tonic–clonic seizures several times a month, but also had absences again. Lamotrigine was tried, but it increased her seizure frequency and topiramate was effective, but she developed paranoia and had to switch. A vagus nerve stimulator was implanted, which reduced the absences and generalized seizures by 50%. Levetiracetam and clobazam were also tried, but the refractory situation continued. During this time, she had to have a personal assistant and could not work. Unfortunately, she developed pancreatic cancer in 2003 and died of the cancer and not of epilepsy in 2004.

General remarks

When a patient is seizure free, the physician needs to be very careful when considering switching drugs even if the particular drug is not necessarily the "best one" recommended. After experiencing the refractoriness of this patient, I am very wary of altering therapies unless there is a very good and solid reason for it. Particularly in syndromes such as absence with generalized tonic–clonic seizures, seizures will occur when stopping a drug and even switching, as we can see from this patient, and can be precarious. Seizures after a period of seizure freedom may become refractory and result in a catastrophic change in the quality of life.

Suggested reading

Ramos-Lizana J, Aquirre-Rodriquez J, Aquilera-Lopez P, Cassinello- Garcia E. Recurrence risk after withdrawal of antiepileptic drugs in children with epilepsy: a prospective study. *Eur J Paediatr Neurol* 2010; 14: 16–24.

Case Studies in Epilepsy, ed. Hermann Stefan, Elinor Ben-Menachem, Patrick Chauvel and Renzo Guerrini. Published by Cambridge University Press. © Hermann Stefan, Elinor Ben-Menachem, Patrick Chauvel and Renzo Guerrini 2012.

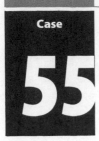

Case

55

Never ever give up

Elinor Ben-Menachem

History

This is a woman who was born in 1948. She is married, has no children, is a heavy smoker and had a sick pension because of lumbago ischias and epilepsy. At the age of nine, she had some kind of meningitis or encephalitis, but the history is not really clear. Her first generalized tonic–clonic seizure occurred in 1967 at the age of 19 and she went on to have many GTCs and seizures that were classified as absences. She was given the usual medication of that time, which was phenytoin and phenobarbital/primidone, but her seizures continued with several GTCs per month and frequent absences a day. Her EEG in 1973, as well as in 1995, showed bilateral synchronized slow spike and waves without focal origins. During her GTCs she often fell and had multiple fractures. For example, in 1995 she had a toe fracture in her left foot and a radial fracture of her right arm after a single seizure. In 1995 she started to develop sudden falls and this could happen several times a day. These sudden falls could be so violent that she was not able to walk alone and her husband had to either hold her or she had to sit in a wheelchair. Her last injury (fractured jaw) was in 2008 because of an atonic attack.

This patient had tried every drug available over the years (phenobarbital, phenytoin, primidone, valproate, carbamazepine, clobazam, clonazepam) and the newer ones that were tried to no avail were gabapentin (no effect), lamotrigine (worsening), topiramate (slow thinking and no effect on seizures), zonisamide (no effect) and levetiracetam (no convincing effect), but she still continues. Finally, in 2008 in total desperation after her jaw

fracture, she was prescribed rufinamide because of the slight chance that it might affect her atonic seizures even if she was not a patient with the diagnosis of Lennox–Gastaut, since rufinamide is an orphan drug for that indication. Also, she had severe osteoporosis probably due to the years on phenytoin–primidone therapy, which could never be reduced without risk to seizure aggravation. Rufinamide was prescribed at the beginning of 2009 and she reached a dose of 2400 mg, which is the normal dose for an adult. The seizures became remarkably better for the first time in her life, but she developed a slight rash and was very dizzy. Trying to weigh the side effects and balance them with the fact that she was almost seizure free for the first time since she was 19, rufinamide was reduced reluctantly to 2000 mg/day. This was still too high because she fell when dizzy (says it was not a seizure) and actually hit her head and suffered a subarachnoidal bleed. This was, of course, just as dangerous as having seizures, so we reduced her rufinamide down to 1200 mg. Since then, she feels that she tolerates the drug and has had no further side effects. She is not now entirely seizure free, but her drop attacks have stopped and so have her generalized tonic–clonic seizures, and she has just had a few absences during the last year. Her husband is much older than she is and now he has serious osteoporosis and needs her help to get around.

The patient is also being treated for osteoporosis and hopefully she will not have another fracture. Unfortunately, attempts to reduce her phenytoin treatment are filled with hazards, and we have been afraid, at this stage, to change her other medications.

Case Studies in Epilepsy, ed. Hermann Stefan, Elinor Ben-Menachem, Patrick Chauvel and Renzo Guerrini. Published by Cambridge University Press. © Hermann Stefan, Elinor Ben-Menachem, Patrick Chauvel and Renzo Guerrini 2012.

General remarks

The patient in these last two cases had seemingly primary generalized seizures but were not easily treated with the recommended drugs for the seizure types we think they had. What we can learn is that, however difficult the diagnosis or treatment, patients today can hope for a better life and there is even hope for many patients to become seizure free even if it may take years. It is easy to be pessimistic and say that once a patient has tried two or more AEDs, then he is refractory and no effort with other AEDs need be undertaken. These two patients prove that this is not the case, and even if they had to suffer from frequent seizures most of their lives, their future was bright and their reliance on the health care system is now much reduced, which is a saving for all.

Special remarks

Osteoporosis is a subject that should not be forgotten when treating patients, both men and especially women who tend to have a higher occurrence of osteoporosis even in the normal population. The patient in this case study should have been treated with calcium and vitamin D from the start. However, this relationship with phenytoin and osteoporosis was not known in the 1950s–1980s. She was given calcium, but only in 1995. However, if possible, one should try to choose drugs that do not cause osteoporosis, which might not be so easy since we do not know exactly which ones they are. There is documentation, however, that phenytoin, carbamazepine, phenobarbital, and valproate are implicated.

Suggested reading

Lee RH, Lyles KW, Colon-Emeric C. A review of the effect of anticonvulsant medications on bone mineral density and fracture risk. *Am J Geriatr Pharmacother* 2010; 8: 34–46.

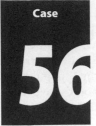

Case

Hippocampal deep brain stimulation may be an alternative for resective surgery in medically refractory temporal lobe epilepsy

Mathieu Sprengers, Paul Boon, and Kristl Vonck

Clinical history

A 33-year-old man who had been suffering from seizures for 21 years, presented at our hospital for a second opinion. Apart from two head injuries at the age of 8 months and 11 years, he had no relevant medical history. There was no family history of neurological or other diseases.

His seizures are preceded by an epigastric rising sensation followed by motionless stare with impaired consciousness. During the past year he has reported a mean seizure frequency of about eight complex partial seizures per week. Once per week he experiences a secondary generalized tonic–clonic seizure. Antiepileptic drugs (phenytoin, carbamazepine, clonazepam and lamotrigine) have failed to significantly decrease the seizure frequency.

Clinical examination

Apart from gingival hyperplasia due to long-term treatment with phenytoin, the clinical and neurological examination was strictly normal.

Technical investigations – presurgical evalution

The patient was enrolled in a presurgical evaluation protocol and underwent the following investigations to identify the epileptogenic zone:

- MRI of the brain: bilateral decreased signal in the area of the dentate gyrus and the cornu ammonis on inversion recovery T1-weighted images without clear lateralization; volume and signal of both hippocampi were normal;
- Interictal FDG-PET scan: hypometabolic zone in the left anterior temporal lobe;

- Video–scalp EEG monitoring: seven recorded seizures showed ictal onset in the left temporal lobe (with secondary generalization in three out of seven seizures)
- Neuropsychological assessment revealed a TIQ of 127 and suggested the presence of a marked right mesotemporal dysfunction.

Conclusion

Video–EEG monitoring and the interictal FDG-PET scan were compatible with localization-related epilepsy with onset in the left temporal lobe. However, the MRI demonstrated no clear lateralization and the neuropsychological evaluation showed a right mesotemporal dysfunction.

During the multidisciplinary epilepsy surgery meeting, it was decided to perform additional investigations:

- WADA test: after injection of amobarbital in the right carotid artery, a left-sided memory score of 6/11 was obtained; left carotid artery injection resulted in a right-sided memory score of 7/11; the patient had a left-hemispheric language dominance;
- Functional MRI confirmed a left-hemispheric language dominance.

These investigations support potential candidacy of this patient for a left-sided temporal lobe invasive procedure. Due to the absence of an identifiable structural lesion on MRI and in the presence of contradicting noninvasive investigation (neuropsychological testing) in a patient with a somewhat atypical medical history of refractory complex partial seizures, it was decided to perform invasive video–EEG monitoring to define the epileptic focus more precisely. Bilateral amygdalohippocampal depth electrodes, a left-sided neocortical grid,

Case Studies in Epilepsy, ed. Hermann Stefan, Elinor Ben-Menachem, Patrick Chauvel and Renzo Guerrini. Published by Cambridge University Press. © Hermann Stefan, Elinor Ben-Menachem, Patrick Chauvel and Renzo Guerrini 2012.

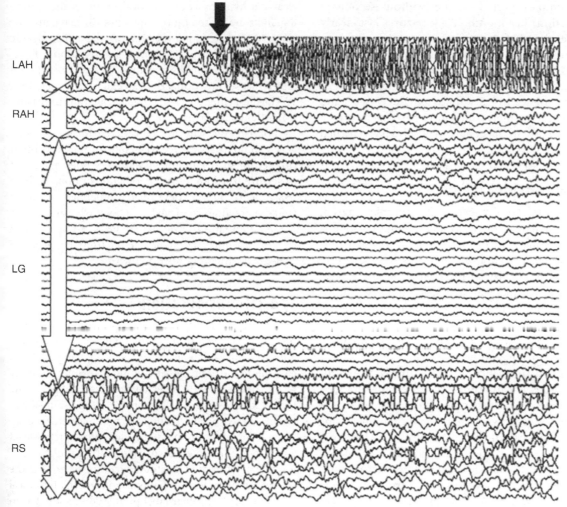

Fig. 1. Intracranial EEG recording of a habitual seizure showing a focal left-sided amygdalohippocampal seizure onset (↓). LAH: left-sided amygdalohippocampal electrode contacts; RAH: right-sided amygdalohippocampal electrode contacts; LG: left-sided neocortical temporal grid contacts; RS: right-sided neocortical temporal strip electrode contact.

and a right-sided neocortical strip were implanted. This invasive monitoring session allowed recording of four habitual seizures and localized the ictal onset zone in the left hippocampus (see Fig. 1).

Diagnosis

Localization-related epilepsy with onset in the left hippocampus in the absence of a clear anatomic correlate on MRI.

Treatment and follow-up

At the end of the presurgical evaluation, the patient was offered resective surgery with chances of becoming seizure free estimated to be around 60%, which is clearly less compared to a typical hippocampal sclerosis case. As an alternative, the patient was offered the opportunity to participate in an ongoing clinical trial with hippocampal deep brain stimulation (DBS). After a trial of 14 days of unilateral left-sided stimulation with the generator still externalized at an output voltage of 1 V, a pulse width of 450 µs, and a pulse frequency of 130 Hz, the patient responded well showing a >50% reduction of the interictal spikes. He then entered the chronic deep brain stimulation phase of the study. After implantation of the pulse generator, his seizure frequency was reduced almost immediately by more than 90% to a mean seizure frequency

173

of one complex partial seizure (without secondary generalization) per month. These seizures last clearly less longer than before DBS treatment and are sometimes confined to a mere aura without obvious loss of consciousness. Association of new antiepileptic drugs (levetiracetam and lacosamide) and augmentation of the output voltage to 2.5 V failed to reduce his seizure frequency any further. The patient has experienced a marked increase in his quality of life and has returned to gainful employment.

General considerations

Localization-related epilepsy with complex partial seizures originating in the (mesial) temporal lobe is the most frequent form of medically refractory epilepsy in adults. The aura preceding this type of seizure varies from an epigastric rising sensation, the experience of déjà-vu and fear to visual, auditory, and/or olfactory hallucinations. Complex partial seizures are characterized by manual and/or orobuccal automatisms, motionless stare, language problems, unilateral dystonic posturing, and head version.

When two (in theory) or more (in practice) antiepileptic drugs fail to render the patient seizure free, other therapeutic strategies should be considered. The first option is resective surgery (temporal lobectomy, selective amygdalohippocampectomy or temporal lesionectomy). Today, this is the most efficacious and evidence-based therapy for medically refractory temporal lobe epilepsy, with seizure freedom being achieved in 50% to 65% of patients at 5 to 10 years of follow-up. The best results are obtained in patients with hippocampal sclerosis, the most common cause of refractory temporal lobe epilepsy. However, resective surgery is only a treatment option when (1) the epileptogenic zone can be identified accurately; and (2) there is no overlap between the epileptogenic zone and the eloquent cortex. In order to evaluate these two criteria, patients are enrolled in a presurgical evaluation protocol. A first evaluation consists of a video–scalp EEG monitoring, 3T structural MRI, interictal FDG-PET scan and a neuropsychological assessment. When the results of these investigations are not fully congruent, additional non-invasive (MEG source localization, ictal SPECT) and invasive video–EEG monitoring may be indicated. The ultimate gold standard to identify the epileptogenic zone is invasive video–EEG monitoring. However, this is an invasive procedure that should only be performed, based on a

clear-cut hypothesis on the localization of the epileptogenic zone (based on previous non-invasive investigations). Besides identification of the epileptogenic zone by the above-mentioned investigations, functional overlap should be excluded. In case of temporal lobe epilepsy, functional overlap can be evaluated by a WADA test (memory and language lateralization) and fMRI (language lateralization).

For patients who are considered unsuitable surgery candidates, who feel reluctant to undergo brain surgery, or in whom epilepsy surgery does not result in seizure freedom, other therapeutic options include trials with newly developed antiepileptic drugs (seizure freedom achieved in about 6%) and vagus nerve stimulation. The latter leads to a marked (>50%) seizure frequency reduction in 50% of patients during long-term follow-up.

Special considerations

Deep brain stimulation is another, however still experimental, treatment strategy for epilepsy. This therapy aims to reduce or abolish seizures by applying electrical currents to the brain, either continuously/intermittently or only in response to detected electrical changes in the brain ("closed-loop" or "responsive" deep brain stimulation). Based on the stimulated brain structure, deep brain stimulation can be subdivided into (1) ictal-onset zone; and (2) remote network structure stimulation.

The most frequently studied ictal-onset zone is the mesial temporal lobe in patients with mesial temporal lobe epilepsy. An open-label pilot study conducted in our center (Reference Center for Refractory Epilepsy, Ghent University Hospital, Belgium) showed encouraging results. After a mean follow-up of 8½ years, 3/11 patients were seizure free for more than 3 years, 3/11 patients (including the patient presented here) had a ≥ 90% reduction in seizure frequency, 3/11 had a moderate response with a seizure frequency reduction of 40%–70% and 2/11 patients were nonresponders. Combining these outcomes with those found in four other studies results in a mean seizure frequency reduction of 59% with a 71% responder rate (i.e., ≥ 50% seizure frequency reduction).

Epileptic network structure stimulation is another approach. Various intracranial targets have been studied, including the anterior and centromedian thalamic nucleus, the cerebellum, the subthalamic nucleus and the caudate nucleus. Anterior thalamic nucleus deep brain stimulation (the most frequently studied remote network structure) resulted in a mean seizure frequency reduction of 54% in five small open trials (63% responders) and a median 56% reduction (54% responders) after 2 years in a large RCT (SANTE-trial).

Future perspectives

Current evidence for clinical efficacy of deep brain stimulation in refractory epilepsy is based mainly on open-label pilot studies and on small double-blind clinical trials. In the future, larger randomized controlled clinical trials are required in order to confirm the promising results and to determine the most efficacious stimulation target and protocol. Furthermore, more research is necessary to unravel the mechanism of action of deep brain stimulation for epilepsy.

Suggested reading

Boon P, Vonck K, De Herdt V, et al. Deep brain stimulation in patients with refractory temporal lobe epilepsy. Epilepsia 2007; 48: 1551–60.

Carrette E, Vonck K, Boon P. The management of pharmacologically refractory epilepsy. CML. Neurol 2010; 26: 104–21.

de Tisi J, Bell G, Peacock J, et al. The long-term outcome of adult epilepsy surgery, patterns of seizure remission, and relapse: a cohort study. Lancet 2011; 378: 1388–95.

Engel J, Wiebe S, French J, et al. Practice parameter: temporal lobe and localized neocortical resections for epilepsy – Report of the quality standards subcommittee of the American Academy of Neurology, in association with the American Epilepsy Society and the American Association of Neurological Surgeons. Neurology 2003; 60: 538–47.

Fisher R, Salanova V, Witt T, et al. Electrical stimulation of the anterior nucleus of thalamus for treatment of refractory epilepsy. Epilepsia 2010; 51: 899–908.

Hamani C, Andrade D, Hodaie M, et al. Deep brain stimulation for the treatment of epilepsy. Int J. Neural Syst 2009; 19: 213–26.

Lega BC, Halpern HH, Jaggi JL, et al. Deep brain stimulation in the treatment of refractory epilepsy: update on current data and future directions. Neurobiol Dis 2010; 38: 354–60.

Morrell MJ, RSES Grp. Responsive cortical stimulation for the treatment of medically intractable partial epilepsy. Neurology 2011; 77: 1295–304.

Ryvlin P, Rheims P. Epilepsy surgery: eligibility criteria and presurgical evaluation. Dialogues Clin Neurosci 2008; 10: 91–103.

Vonck K, Boon P, Achten E, et al. Long-term amygdalohippocampal stimulation for refractory temporal lobe epilepsy. Ann. Neurol 2002; 52: 556–65.

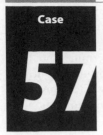

Case 57

Myoclonic seizures and recurrent nonconvulsive status epilepticus in Dravet syndrome

Francesco Mari and Renzo Guerrini

Clinical history

A 3-year-old female patient with Dravet syndrome was brought to our attention due to episodes of absences with myoclonic jerks and recurrent periods of obtundation states of undetermined etiology.

General history

Her disease history started at age 4 months with prolonged febrile and afebrile hemiclonic seizures. Phenobarbital was initially introduced with transient benefit. After a few months, drug-resistant absences with rhythmic myoclonic jerks occurred. Valproate and clobazam associated with stiripentol were progressively introduced to replace phenobarbital with only a transient response. Several neuropsychological evaluations disclosed moderate cognitive impairment. A presumptive diagnosis of Dravet syndrome was confirmed by genetic testing, revealing a *de novo* mutation of the sodium channel α1 subunit gene (*SCN1A*) gene (c.680T<C, Fig. 1).

Examination

Prolonged video–EEG monitoring captured frequent, brief episodes of myoclonic absences (Fig. 2) and periods of obtundation, which proved to be episodes of nonconvulsive status (Fig. 3). Ethosuximide was introduced and stiripentol was withdrawn. Episodes of nonconvulsive status episodes persisted, but were subsequently controlled and went under persistent remission after a cycle of hydrocortisone treatment.

Image findings

Brain MRI was normal.

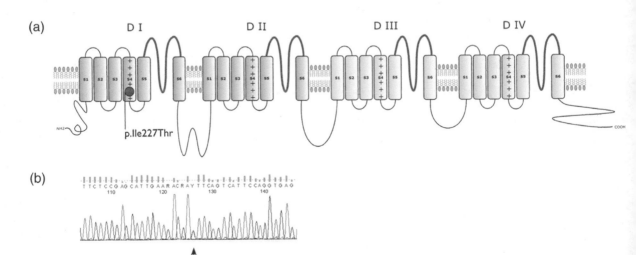

Fig. 1. Schematic drawing representing the transmembrane location of the aminoacidic change resulting from the c.680T>C change.

Case Studies in Epilepsy, ed. Hermann Stefan, Elinor Ben-Menachem, Patrick Chauvel and Renzo Guerrini. Published by Cambridge University Press. © Hermann Stefan, Elinor Ben-Menachem, Patrick Chauvel and Renzo Guerrini 2012.

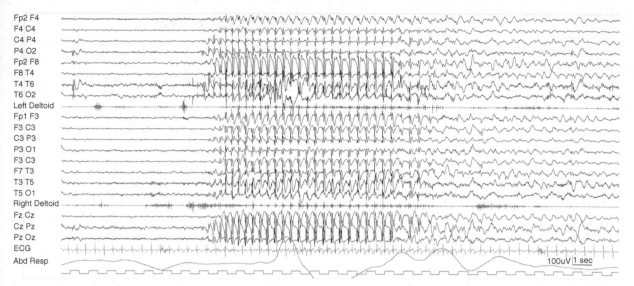

Fig. 2. Video–EEG recording: myoclonic absence episode related to bilateral spikes and polyspikes and wave discharges. The EMG channels (left deltoid, right deltoid) show rhythmic myoclonic bursts temporally related to the spike component of spike and wave discharges.

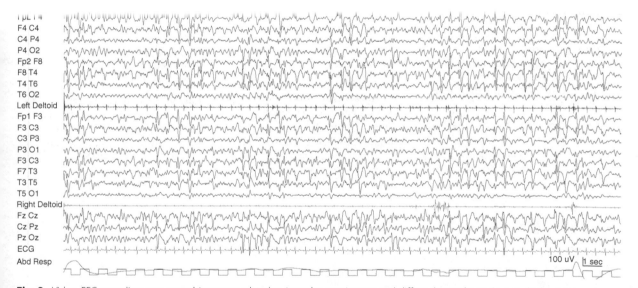

Fig. 3. Video–EEG recording: non-convulsive status related to irregular, continuous, and diffuse slow spike and wave discharges.

Follow-up

At age 5 years, the patient exhibits moderate cognitive impairment and daily myoclonic absences. Her EEG shows multifocal paroxysmal abnormalities.

Diagnosis

Recurrent nonconvulsive status epilepticus, and myoclonic absences in a patient with Dravet syndrome.

General remarks

Dravet syndrome is an epileptic encephalopathy with onset in the first year of life. The clinical picture is characterized, at onset, by repeated and prolonged generalized or unilateral, clonic or tonic–clonic seizures precipitated by fever. Subsequently, afebrile drug-resistant seizures appear of variable semiology, including atypical absence, myoclonic, and focal. Mutations of the *SCN1A* gene, mostly *de novo* are found in about 80% of patients. About 5% of patients exhibit genomic rearrangements involving the *SCN1A* gene. These patients would result mutation negative if tested with traditional Sanger sequencing. In most patients, after epilepsy onset, cognitive and behavioral hyperactivity become apparent, with most patients showing progressive slowing of acquired skills.

Special remarks

Pharmacological approach to patients with Dravet Syndrome is challenging. Phenobarbital, valproate, topiramate, and benzodiazepines have been used with some results. Stiripentol, associated with clobazam, has been shown to be effective in two double-blind, randomized trials. Phenytoin, carbamazepine, and lamotrigine should be avoided as they have been reported to precipitate seizure worsening.

Future perspectives

In a small percentage of female patients with a phenotype reminiscent of Dravet syndrome, mutations in protocadherin 19 (*PCDH19*) gene have been reported. Similarities relate more to the precipitating role of fever than to seizure types, as most girls with *PCDH19* mutations have focal seizures. In about 10% of patients the etiology remains unknown. Differences in phenotype severity, even within the same family, suggest that a permissive genetic background may influence the expression of the disorder. Animal models have been instrumental in demonstrating that loss of function in GABAergic interneurons is the basis for hyperexcitability of pyramidal neurons as the underlying basis for epileptogenesis. It has been shown that specific folding defective mutants can be rescued by interactions with associated proteins and drugs in vivo. Modulating the effect of the mutation in vivo influences the phenotype. Interacting drugs may be used to rescue the mutant in vivo.

Suggested reading

Catarino CB, Liu JY, Liagkouras I, *et al*. Dravet syndrome as epileptic encephalopathy: evidence from long-term course and neuropathology. *Brain* 2011; **134**: 2982–3010.

Dravet C. The core Dravet syndrome phenotype. *Epilepsia* 2011; **52**: 3–9.

Dravet C. Dravet syndrome history. *Dev Med Child Neurol* 2011; **53**: 1–6.

Guerrini R, Dravet C, Genton P, *et al*. Lamotrigine and seizure aggravation in severe myoclonic epilepsy. *Epilepsia* 1998; **39**: 508–12.

Marini C, Mei D, Parmeggiani L, *et al*. Protocadherin 19 mutations in girls with infantile-onset epilepsy. *Neurology* 2010; **75**: 646–53.

Marini C, Scheffer IE, Nabbout R, *et al*. The genetics of Dravet syndrome. *Epilepsia* 2011; **52**: 24–9.

Ragona F, Granata T, Dalla Bernardina B, *et al*. Cognitive development in Dravet syndrome: a retrospective, multicenter study of 26 patients. *Epilepsia* 2011; **52**: 386–92.

Rusconi R, Scalmani P, Cassulini RR, *et al*. Modulatory proteins can rescue a trafficking defective epileptogenic Nav1.1 Na$^+$ channel mutant. *J Neurosci* 2007; **27**: 11037–46.

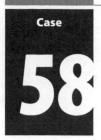

Case

58 Functional hemispherotomy for drug-resistant post-traumatic epilepsy

Francesco Mari and Renzo Guerrini

Clinical history

An 11-year-old boy was admitted to our ward for evaluation of a severe form of symptomatic focal epilepsy.

General history

At age 2 years, a severe head injury had occurred in relation to a road accident, with acute subdural hematoma and residual left hemiparesis and hemianopia.

At age 5 years, focal motor seizures appeared that rapidly reached a daily frequency and proved drug resistant.

Examination

Neurological examination on admission: left hemiparesis and hemianopia, moderate hyperactivity, and aggressive behavior.

Prolonged video–EEG recordings revealed frequent bilateral and mostly asynchronous interictal abnormalities and captured several seizures with asymmetric tonic posturing, mainly involving the right hemibody (Fig. 1(a),(b)).

Previous neuroimaging had documented severe atrophy of the right brain hemisphere with bilateral subcortical lesions in the frontal lobes (Fig. 2).

Special studies

Through i.v. infusion of benzodiazepines during continuous EEG recording, we confirmed that interictal paroxysmal activity was lateralized to the right (Fig. 1(c)).

Follow-up

We performed a vertical paramedian functional hemispherotomy. At 31 months of follow-up, the patient is seizure free. Striking improvement of cognitive and behavioral skills has occurred (Fig. 3(a)).

Image findings

Presurgery MRI: (Fig. 2).

Postoperative MRI: highlights the extent and trajectory of the neurosurgical approach (Fig. 3).

Diagnosis

Drug-resistant post-traumatic lateralized multilobar epilepsy

General remarks

Disconnection procedures are considered to represent an effective treatment option for intractable epilepsy originating from a damaged hemisphere. Hemimegalencephaly, post-traumatic epilepsy, Sturge–Weber syndrome, and Rasmussen encephalitis are typical conditions in which hemispherotomy/hemispherectomy has been widely used. The procedures cause an expected contralateral motor and visual deficit. This drawback is, however, acceptable in patients with pre-existing stable or progressive deficit of these functions. The timing of surgery is an important issue as an earlier approach is correlated with better chances of recovery of function in relation to brain plasticity.

Special remarks

This case report indicates that an older age and the imaging finding of bilateral brain lesions and bilateral interictal EEG discharges should not be considered a contraindication *per se*.

Case Studies in Epilepsy, ed. Hermann Stefan, Elinor Ben-Menachem, Patrick Chauvel and Renzo Guerrini. Published by Cambridge University Press. © Hermann Stefan, Elinor Ben-Menachem, Patrick Chauvel and Renzo Guerrini 2012.

(a)

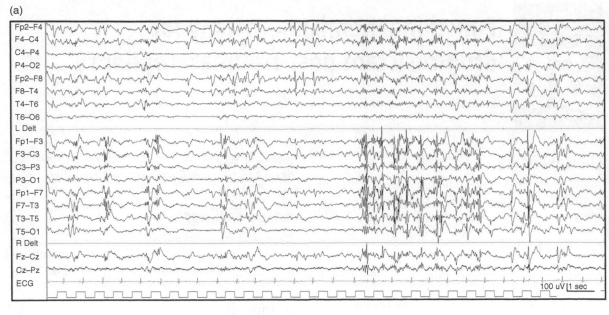

(b)

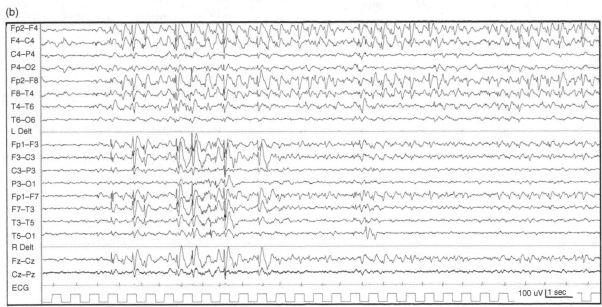

Fig. 1. Prolonged video–EEG recording: interictal bilateral paroxysmal abnormalities (a)(b); EEG after i.v. BDZ revealed right hemispheric predominance of EEG discharges persisting upon infusion (c).

Future perspectives

Improvement of modern and less invasive disconnection techniques, such as vertical paramedian functional hemispherotomy, will reduce the morbidity associated with both functional and anatomical hemispherotomy (hydrocephalus and worsening of hemiparesis). Increased public awareness of this surgical procedure and reduced technical aggressiveness will likely determine an increase in the number of patients operated.

(c)

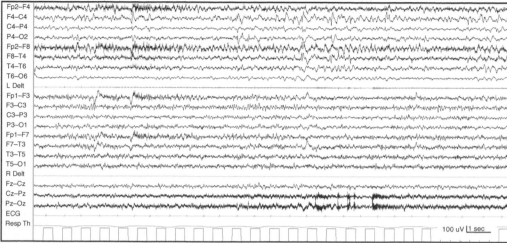

Fig. 1. (*cont.*)

(a)(i)

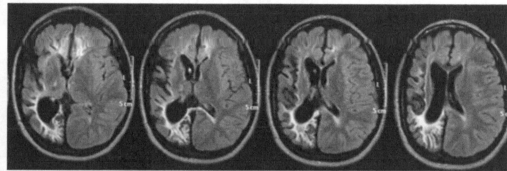

(a)(ii)

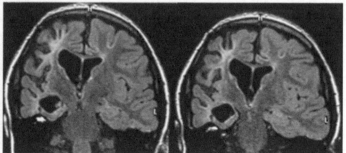

(b)

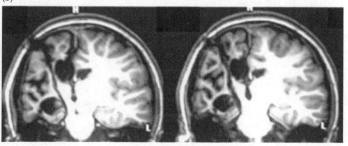

Fig. 2. FLAIR MRI: preoperative scan (a): axial section in the top row and coronal sections in the bottom row. Diffuse cortical and subcortical atrophy of the right hemisphere; abnormal high signal intensity in the white matter of the left frontal lobe. Postoperative examination (b), T1W coronal section showing the trajectory of neurosurgical approach.

181

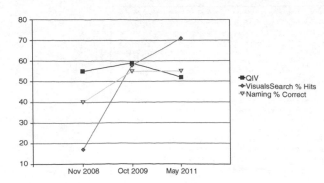

Fig. 3. Serial neuropsychological evaluations.

Suggested reading

Boshuisen K, van Schooneveld MM, Leijten FS, *et al*. Contralateral MRI abnormalities affect seizure and cognitive outcome after hemispherectomy. *Neurology* 2010; **75**: 1623–30.

Caraballo R, Bartuluchi M, Cersosimo R, Soraru A, Pomata H. Hemispherectomy in pediatric patients with epilepsy: a study of 45 cases with special emphasis on epileptic syndromes. *Childs Nerv Syst* 2011; **27**: 2131–6.

Cook SW, Nguyen ST, Hu B, *et al*. Cerebral hemispherectomy in pediatric patients with epilepsy: comparison of three techniques by pathological substrate in 115 patients. *J Neurosurg (Pediatrics 2)* 2004; **100**: 125–141.

De Ribaupierre S, Delalande O. Hemispherotomy and other disconnective techniques. *Neurosurg Focus* 2008; **25**: 1–10.

Pharmacoresistant epilepsy?

59

Tobias Knieß

Clinical history

A 23-year-old woman was admitted to hospital for syndrome classification and therapy optimization because of persistent tonic–clonic, myoclonis, aurac, and disruptions of consciousness lasting short periods (seconds) under the medication of 2000 mg levetiracetam.

General history

A first bilaterally convulsive seizure and myoclonic events occurred 1 year ago after a common cold.

Diagnosis: epilepsy with tonic–clonic, especially Janz' syndrome.

In earlier history, multiple syncopal events and febrile convulsions in childhood.

Application of lamotrigine therapy 200 mg after first seizure; increasing number of seizures and transition to levetiracetam 2000 mg. Continued increase in seizure frequency. Her state examination in ergotherapy had to be postponed twice due to tiredness. Until 2 years ago very good student, then sudden slump in performance due to significant difficulties with concentration and memory. Mother of 4-year-old child. Lives alone. Mother and grandmother provide intensive support.

No other illnesses. No regular consumption of alcohol. No drugs.

Examination

Internal and neurological examination results: unremarkable, left-handed patient.

Psychiatric/psychological findings: evidence of cognitive deficits, psychomotor retardation, vigilance and concentration deficits.

Special studies

Laboratory including drug screening and cortisol: normal findings.

HLA typization: HLA DR 15 and HLA DQ 5 and 6: positive.

Three-day MRA with contrasting agents and temporal lobe angulated thin layer: no morphological brain lesions, no dysplasia, no Ammon's horn sclerosis, no cavernome, no migration disruptions.

Resting wake EEG with *HV* and *TS*: after 2 minutes K-complexes and sleep spindle

Sleep deprivation EEG: *POST*s and K-complexes from beginning of recording.

Video–EEG monitoring under 2000 mg LEV: no epileptic activity. One incident to be noted: after waking up the patient at 6 pm, she was not able to properly communicate, could not speak, seemed disoriented for a duration of 3–4 minutes. Afterwards, psychomotor slowing, but fully oriented. Left arm not responsive for over 14 minutes with increased tonus. Slight shaking on attempts to move hand. No pathological correlate in EEG. During 24 hours of recording, patient was sleeping for 19 hours.

Long-term ECG: sinus rhythm.

Blood glucose day profile: normal.

Schellong test: no evidence for orthostatic dysregulation.

Psychosomatic council: no secure diagnosis and evidence for dissociative seizures.

Neuropsychological diagnosis: attentive and speed performance far below average. Memory deficits, executive abilities impaired.

Follow-up

During her entire stay, the patient was suffering from a noticeable, markedly increased, need for sleep. It was

---

Case Studies in Epilepsy, ed. Hermann Stefan, Elinor Ben-Menachem, Patrick Chauvel and Renzo Guerrini. Published by Cambridge University Press. © Hermann Stefan, Elinor Ben-Menachem, Patrick Chauvel and Renzo Guerrini 2012.

very difficult to wake her and it took 1–5 minutes before she became fully conscious. She nearly fell asleep during the examination of neuropsychological testing.

Additional family history: her mother suffers from a sleep disorder; the reason is unknown to the patient.

She was sent for polysomnography at a co-operating clinic due to suspected sleep disorder (narcolepsy or idiopathic hypersomnia).

Diagnosis

Narcolepsy.

General remarks

Assumed pharmacoresistant epilepsy leads to the early consideration of other possible reasons or non-epileptic seizures. A very important factor is a detailed self and third-party anamnesis under consideration of seemingly irrelevant secondary symptoms. A differentiated supplementary diagnosis such as a video–EEG monitoring is definitely necessary in case of missing seizure-free periods and not certainly classified epilepsy. Narcolepsy does not have to be associated with cataplectic seizures (monosymptomatic narcolepsy). The disability of the left arm and the impaired speech after awakening correspond mostly with a partial involvement or with a sleep paralysis. To confirm the diagnosis, a HLA typecast (HLA DR 15 and HLA DQ5 and 6) should be performed. Another significant marker is the identification of hypocretin in the brain fluid.

Future perspectives

Levetiracetam was discontinued, and modafinil therapy initiated; genetical diagnosis with hypocretin in brain fluid initiated. Neuropsychological follow-ups are recommended after 6 months. Driver's license has been suspended until further notice. The state examination has to be postponed until after recovery.

Progression

No further seizure-like incidents occurred during modafinil therapy.

Vagus nerve stimulation for epilepsy

60

Barbara Schmalbach and Nicolas Lang

Clinical history

A 19-year-old female patient with a medical history of depression, personality disorder, and obesity presented to our epilepsy outpatient department with uncontrolled simple and complex partial seizures. The patient's history of seizures began at the age of 16, when she experienced episodes of vertigo and blurred vision accompanied by a sense of colored spots and followed by staring, fidgeting, lip smacking, and impairment of awareness as well as amnesia for the seizures. These episodes lasted 10–60 seconds and occurred three times per week at time of presentation. The seizures seemed to be provoked by stressful situations and contact with hot water.

General history

Depression, personality disorder, and obesity with a Body Mass Index (BMI) of 36.8.

Examination

On neurological examination, there was no evidence for other neurological or psychiatric deficits.

Special studies

Brain MRI showed bilateral left accentuated cortical band heterotopias, ranging from frontal to occipital with a perinsular diameter of 4 mm in coronal sections (Fig. 1). Interictal surface EEG showed intermittent left fronto-temporal slowing. Video–EEG monitoring for 48 hours showed interictally intermittent bilateral temporal and right frontal spikes as well as intermittent bilateral left accentuated temporal slowing. Furthermore, three clinically apparent seizures with correlates in the EEG occurred with bifrontal slowing, followed by right hemispheric

slowing with right frontal accentuation and intermittend right frontal sharp waves for 50 seconds.

Follow-up

For the first few years from the onset of seizures, numerous regimens of antiepileptic drugs were tried without beneficial long-term effects. The antiepileptic drugs either led to no substantial benefit or provoked intolerable adverse effects. Oxcarbazepine led to aggressive behavior, valproate had to be stopped due to massive weight gain, and zonisamide increased memory problems. After a brief trial with oxcarbazepine in monotherapy, it was given with varying combinations of lamotrigine, valproate, zonisamide, and topiramate. Subsequently, under a combination of lamotrigine and topiramate, seizure frequency was ameliorated, but the situation concerning seizures and especially quality of life was not satisfying. Since the patient seemed to be refractory to antiepileptic drugs, she was referred to an epilepsy center for

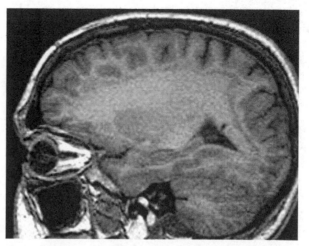

Fig. 1. Subcortical band heterotopias along the fronto-occiptal axis.

Case Studies in Epilepsy, ed. Hermann Stefan, Elinor Ben-Menachem, Patrick Chauvel and Renzo Guerrini. Published by Cambridge University Press. © Hermann Stefan, Elinor Ben-Menachem, Patrick Chauvel and Renzo Guerrini 2012.

presurgical evaluation, but the lesion did not turn out to be operable. This was why the decision for implantation of a vagus nerve stimulator (VNS) was made. After implantation, seizure frequency was significantly reduced and auras could be interrupted by manually activating stimulation with the magnet at the first sign or warning of an impending seizure. Finally, quality of life markedly improved.

Diagnosis

Focal epilepsy with simple and complex partial seizures due to bilateral subcortical band heterotopias.

General remarks

Approximately one-third of patients with epilepsy suffer from refractory seizures, despite optimal antiepileptic drug (AED) therapy, or else they experience unacceptable side effects.

There is broad evidence that, for patients with partial-onset seizures, who are not seizure free despite numerous regimens of antiepileptic drugs and who are not considered as appropriate candidates for resective epilepsy surgery, vagus nerve stimulation (VNS) is an appropriate alternative option. VNS also seems to be effective in patients with other seizure types.

Around one-third of patients benefit from a treatment with VNS, i.e., they show a 50% or greater reduction in seizures; however, the number of patients reaching a 50% seizure reduction seems to increase with time. On the other hand, only few patients achieve freedom from seizures and almost all remain on AEDs. Not only does seizure frequency respond to stimulation in some patients, but also mood, memory, and quality of life seem to improve under therapy with VNS, which is reflected by low withdrawal rates. However, this therapy is considered palliative and is reserved for patients who are not candidates for surgery or for whom surgery has failed. So far, it has not been possible to predict which patients will benefit from VNS. Improvement is not immediate, but tends to increase over 18–24 months of treatment.

One advantage of VNS is the missing cognitive side effect often noticeable with increasing doses of antiepileptic drugs. VNS side effects are confined to cough, voice alteration, and hoarseness as well as a feeling of tightness or even pain in the throat area, which are mainly stimulation related, reversible, and tend to diminish with time. Mild to moderate symptoms of vomiting, dyspnea and paresthesias have also been reported. Caution is necessary when patients undergo MRI.

In order to implant a VNS, a simple extracranial neurosurgical operation is necessary during which a device consisting of a pulse generator similar to a cardiac pacemaker is implanted subcutaneously under the left clavicle, and a lead wire consisting of two helical bipolar stimulating electrodes is tunnelled under the skin and placed around the left vagus nerve. The generator is programmed using a telemetry wand held over the device, with settings for current intensity, pulse width, and frequency. Time on stimulation is typically 30–90 seconds and is followed by 3 to 5 minutes off stimulation with a cycling of 24 hours/day. The times on and off can be altered, and many clinicians use rapid cycling of 7 seconds on and 0,2 seconds off, but there is no evidence that any time setting is better than another and the optimum stimulation parameters are still unknown. In addition to a continuous stimulation mode, the device can be activated manually at the first sign or warning of an impending seizure by a magnet swiped over the skin where the stimulator is implanted. Complication rates of the operation are low and include infections, vocal cord paresis, lower facial weakness, bradycardia, and asystole.

The mechanism of action is not fully understood; current information suggests that VNS activates neuronal networks in the thalamus and other limbic structures, and that norepinephrine may mediate the antiseizure activity of VNS.

Future perspectives

There is preliminary evidence that VNS might be effective in patients with less refractory epilepsy and this may be the future use of VNS. However, more research is needed to provide evidence of efficacy in these patients.

Suggested reading

Ben-Menachem E. Vagus nerve stimulation for the treatment of epilepsy. *Lancet Neurol* 2002; **1**: 477–82.

Ben-Menachem E, Manon-Espaillat R, Ristanovic, *et al*. Vagus nerve stimulation for treatment of partial seizures: 1. A controlled study of effect on seizures. *Epilepsia* 1994; **35**: 616–26.

Handforth A, De Georgio CM, Schachter SC, *et al*. Vagus nerve stimulation therapy for partial seizures. A randomized active-control trial. *Neurology* 1998; **51**: 48–55.

Morris GL, Mueller WM. Long-term treatment with vagus nerve stimulation in patients with refractory epilepsy. The Vagus Nerve Stimulation Study Group E01-E05. *Neurology* 1999; **53**: 1731–5.

Case 61

The strange behavior of a vegetarian: a diagnostic indicator for treatment? (a quiz case)

Katrin Hüttemann and Hermann Stefan

Clinical history

A 61-year-old woman visited the canteen with a colleague. The colleague was surprised that the woman ordered a sausage, because normally she was a passionate vegetarian.

Furthermore, the colleague noticed that the woman seemed to be confused that day. Due to this, he took her to a hospital emergency room.

General history

The patient was a healthy woman with no mentionable history.

Examination

The patient was slightly disorientated without any focal neurological deficit. She had no history of any previous epileptic seizures.

Question to the reader

1. Which investigations should be carried out as a minimum:
   - blood sugar?
   - cerebrospinal fluid ?
   - EEG ?
   - MRI ?
   - cognitive testing ?
   - liver function testing ?
2. What is the presumed diagnosis?

Diagnosis

Non-convulsive status epilepticus.

Case Studies in Epilepsy, ed. Hermann Stefan, Elinor Ben-Menachem, Patrick Chauvel and Renzo Guerrini. Published by Cambridge University Press. © Hermann Stefan, Elinor Ben-Menachem, Patrick Chauvel and Renzo Guerrini 2012.

Results

EEG showed a pattern of continuous generalized 2–3 Hz spike and wave complexes.

MRI and analysis of the cerebral spinal fluid were unremarkable.

After 6 mg of clonazepam, the EEG changed to beta-wave-activity.

Treatment with benzodiazepine and valproic acid was commenced and the patient had no further epileptic seizures.

Non-convulsive status epilepticus is characterized by a clouding of consciousness and behavioral changes for at least 30 minutes with typical EEG findings. In an adult you have to differentiate between a generalized and a partial non-convulsive status epilepticus. In the generalized non-convulsive status you can normally find bilateral diffuse synchronous activity. It has to be assumed that the non-convulsive status is underdiagnosed because,

as in the described patient, the diagnosis is only possible if an EEG is performed. However, this is often one of the problems in the diagnosis because an EEG is often unavailable out of hours or at weekends.

One further problem in the diagnosis is to decide which EEG patterns represent ictal states as opposed to interictal (for example, paroxysmal lateralized epileptiform discharges (PLED) or even physiologic patterns or EEG artifacts.

Typical generalized (absence) status can usually be stopped by intravenous benzodiazepine. Contrary to the convulsive status epilepticus, this is a more benign form of status epilepticus with a better outcome, but nonetheless it should be treated with antiepileptic drugs.

The available data suggest that generalized (absence) status epilepticus does not accompany lasting morbidity.

Suggested reading

Drislane FW. Evidence against permanent neurologic damage from nonconvulsive status epilepticus. *J Clin Neurophysiol* 1999; **16**: 332–40.

Heckmann JG, Lang CJ, Stefan H, Neundörfer B. The vegetarian who ate a sausage with curry sauce. *The Lancet Neurology* 2003; **2**: 62.

Kaplan PW. Assessing the outcomes in patients with nonconvulsive status epilepticus: nonconvulsive status epilepticus is underdiagnosed, potentially overtreated, and confounded by comorbidity. *J Clin Neurohysiol* 1999; **16**: 341–52.

Kaplan PW. Prognosis in nonconvulsive status epilepticus. *Epileptic Disord* 2000; **2**: 1985–94.

Krumholz A. Epidemiology and evidence for morbidity

of nonconvulsive status epilepticus. *J Clin Neurophysiol* 1999; **16**: 332–40.

Scholtes FB, Renier WO, Meinardi H. Non-convulsive status epilepticus: causes, treatment and outcome in 65 patients. *J Neurol Neurosurg Psychiatry* 1996; **61**: 93–5.

Shorvon S. The management of status epilepticus. *J Neurol Neurosurg Psychiatry* 2001; **70**: 22–7.

Index